Designing for
Therapeutic
Environments

Designing for Therapeutic Environments

A Review of Research

Edited by

David Canter

Department of Psychology,
University of Surrey

and

Sandra Canter

Roffey Park Hospital, Sussex
and
Department of Psychology,
University of Surrey

JOHN WILEY & SONS
Chichester · New York · Brisbane · Toronto

British Library Cataloguing in Publication Data:

Designing for therapeutic environments.
   1. Therapeutic community 2. Environmental psychology
 I. Canter, David Victor II. Canter, Sandra
   155.9   RC489.T67   79-40510

ISBN 0 471 27569 7

Printed and bound in Great Britain

Acknowledgments

Bringing together a book of contributions such as the present one depends upon the help and goodwill of a great many people. The idea for this book first saw the light of day as a joint series of seminars presented for the post-graduate courses in Clinical and Environmental Psychology at the University of Surrey. It is partly because of the interest and encouragement of the students that the seminars eventually gave rise to the present book.

We are also grateful to Professor Jack Tizard for his comments on an early draft of the book as well as to Professor Paul Gump for his detailed reading of the original manuscripts.

Finally our thanks to Liz Stephens who produced the camera-ready typescript and to Tony Side who produced the illustrations.

David and Sandra Canter

Notes on Contributors

DAVID CANTER is Director of the Masters course in Environmental Psychology at the University of Surrey. He is author of a number of books, his most recent being "The Psychology of Place".

SANDRA CANTER is a Clinical Psychologist at Roffey Park Hospital and a lecturer in the Department of Psychology at the University of Surrey.

H.C. GUNZBURG, B.A.,M.A.,Ph.D.,F.B.Ps.S., is a Consultant Psychologist at Monyhull Hospital, Birmingham, who developed the "Progress Assessment Chart of Social and Personal Development" (P-A-C). He is Editor of the British Journal of Mental Subnormality.

ANNA L. GUNZBURG, A.R.I.B.,Dip.Ing. (Vienna), is an architect who has worked for many years in educational and health departments and is now a Consultant in mental handicap environmental design. She works in close collaboration with her husband on the provision of stimulating and activating learning programmes.

CHARLES J. HOLAHAN has a Ph.D. in Clinical Psychology from the University of Massachusetts and is currently an assistant professor and associate director of the Community Psychology Program at the University of Texas at Austin.

CHERYL KENNY obtained her bachelors degree in Psychology from the University of California at Berkeley and her M.Sc. in Environmental Psychology at the University of Surrey. She is currently a Research Fellow on the Hospital Evaluation Research Unit at the University of Surrey.

BONNIE KROLL is an Administrative Analyst in the Office for Student Affairs Research and Evaluation at the University of California, Davis.

M. POWELL LAWTON received his doctorate in Clinical Psychology from Columbia University and has been Director of Behavioral Research at the Philadelphia Geriatric Center since 1963. His research has dealt with the environmental psychology of later life.

ALAN LIPMAN has a Personal Chair in Architecture at the
Welsh School of Architecture. He has been an architectural practitioner for some twelve years, has taught
under- and post-graduate courses for fifteen years and
has supervised and conducted architectural and social
science research.

SOPHIA PAPASSOTIRIOU MAZIS is a qualified architect who
completed the M.Sc. in Environmental Psychology at the
University of Surrey. She is a teaching assistant at the
Architectural School of the Aristoteles University of
Thessaloniki.

JOHN RICHER who has an M.A., Ph.D. and Dip.Psych., is now
Senior Clinical Psychologist at the Park Hospital for
Children in Oxford. His main research interest is the
application of human ethology to psychiatric problems,
especially autism.

LEANNE RIVLIN is a member of the Faculty of the Environmental Psychology Program, City University, New York, and
an associate of the Center for Human Environments. She
has studied day care centres, schools and ethnic differences
in space use patterns.

DAVID A. SIME is a Consultant Psychiatrist formerly with
the Devon Area Health Authority in Britain. He has been
actively involved for many years in the areas of mental
handicap and forensic psychiatry. He now works in
Melbourne, Australia.

JONATHAN D. SIME obtained his M.Sc. in Environmental
Psychology from the University of Surrey and is currently
a Research Fellow in the Fire Research Unit at the
University of Surrey.

ROBERT SLATER is a lecturer in the Department of Applied
Psychology at the University of Wales Institute of Science
and Technology. He is a Social Psychologist who teaches
"Human Studies in Architecture" to students at the Welsh
School of Architecture.

ROBERT SOMMER is Professor of Psychology and Director of
the Center for Consumer Research at the University of
California, Davis. His most recent book, "The Mind's Eye",
published by Delta Books in 1978, is concerned with visual
imagery in everyday life.

MAXINE WOLFE is a member of the Faculty of the Environmental Psychology Program, City University, New York, and
an associate of the Center for Human Environments. Her
research interests cover, in addition to institutional
facilities, the study of privacy, environmental experience,
sex roles and spatial ability.

PAUL MARTIN JOHN WOLFF obtained his B.Arch. from the
University of California at Berkeley and his M.Sc. in
Environmental Psychology from the University of Surrey.
He is Associate Professor of Architecture in the School
of Architecture and Environmental Design at California
Polytechnic State University, San Luis Obispo.

Contents

Building for Therapy

SANDRA AND DAVID CANTER

THERAPEUTIC ENVIRONMENTS

In recent years a maturity has become apparent in the views held about the provision of therapeutic environments. After the broadening realization which emerged in the early sixties of the pitfalls and destructive qualities of most institutional settings (Goffman, 1961); after the excitement generated by various attempts at therapeutic communities (Jones, 1952) and community based therapy in many areas of health care provision (Jones, 1962), there was a period of great optimism in the possibility of greatly reducing or removing altogether the number of people who spend long periods of time in large medical or quasi-medical institutions. This optimism coincided with rapid improvement in medical practices, most notably through the use of antibiotics and subsequently the psychotrophic drugs. This change in attitude led to a recognition of the inadequacy of many existing buildings and the determination to use the new-found post war wealth to replace them with modern facilities, appropriate to a wide range of new therapeutic approaches.

This book deals with that emergent concern with building for therapy. It presents evaluations of a range of facilities and provides both an account of the role of the physical environment in therapeutic processes and indicates ways in which physical environments can be more effective.

One unusual aspect of this book, which gives it its main raison d'etre, is that contributions have been deliberately commissioned from people working in as wide a range of therapeutic settings as we could find. In the past,

1

although there have been parallel developments in different
therapeutic areas, there appears to have been no concerted
attempt to bring the various concerns together. Hence, we
have deliberately sought contributions from adult and child
settings, from those where the inmates are psychiatric, handicapped or medically ill, or with the design of a particular
facility such as a playground.

Our aim in doing this has been to show that the problems
and solutions have many common properties across all these
settings. It has also been to demonstrate that difficulties
arise by the naive transference of an approach from one
setting to another. The most commonly recognized of these
difficulties is the transference of the medical approach to
the psychiatric setting, but we believe that the reader will
become aware of many other such inappropriate transfers in
the following pages, either of detail or of policy.

Indeed, perhaps paradoxically, one of the issues which
becomes apparent from comparisons between the various contributions is the importance of relating a design to its
particular therapeutic goals and activities, which typically
involves a careful characterization of the particular
patients. At present there appears to be a great deal of
confusion as to the nature and value of environments designed
for therapy. Architects and the media alike have been
impressed by the possibility of general solutions, whereby
attention to one or two aspects of the design (e.g. a sylvan
setting, a low profile, or plush, colourful furnishings)
have been considered the inevitable generators of a therapeutic environment. The papers in this book demonstrate
that simple fashions can never answer the complex questions
surrounding how therapeutic environments are created. No
one aspect of the provision of therapeutic facilities, be
it drugs, therapists, buildings, or any of those provisions
which are encompassed under the label 'environment', can on
their own produce radically improved services. It is also
apparent that two or more aspects inappropriately put together can drastically reduce the value of the best provision.
A new building with an archaic administrative structure, or
improved hospital facilities without the necessary community
back-up, can lead to a great waste of resources.

This book has been prepared to bring together accounts
of current research and practice. There have been few comparisons of the provisions made for different client groups,
even though there is a surprisingly large area of agreement
between practitioners and researchers who have been concerned
with different populations. In providing this account we

are taking stock of the current situation in Britain and
North America and asking what the real possibilities are for
improvement. We are not concerned with radical solutions
which could only be brought about in special circumstances,
but with the wide range of possibilities which exist at the
present time, their successes and their weaknesses.

What emerges from this account is that there are few
simple answers to these complex issues, but that there is
a great deal which can be done within present day settings
and resources, to greatly improve our therapeutic environments.

It is through the notion of improvement that the term
therapeutic has gained currency. The common definition of
therapy is that which heals (or makes whole), but from its
earliest use it transpires that the word 'therapeuein' has
also meant 'to take care of'. Hence the role of the nurse
(who takes care) and of the physician (who heals) have both
long been accepted as appropriately called therapeutic.

'Environments for therapy' is sometimes taken to mean
places in which therapy occurs: those locations which encap-
sulate therapeutic processes. As such, there may be a
concern with the position in which the facilities are placed,
and possibly with the directly functional requirements to be
met to achieve obvious organisational goals.

A secondary meaning of providing environments for
therapy has been taken as creating situations which will
directly contribute to and enhance any therapeutic processes.
Indeed, some writers such as Cummings and Cummings (1964),
Maxwell Jones (1962) and others have gone to the extreme of
suggesting that the environment is (or ought to be) the
major therapeutic agent in any therapeutic situation. It
can be seen, as a consequence, that the term 'therapeutic
environment' may range in meaning from simply indicating a
location in which takes place various forms of healing and
caring of groups of the population, identified as in some
way unable to cope without the processes provided in the
location; to the more ambitious meaning of a setting which
is itself therapeutic.

Clearly there are many possible gradations between these
two extremes of use of the word 'environment', but to sim-
plify our discussion we will concentrate on the extremes of
this continuum. There are a number of practical considerations which derive from determining to set up a therapeutic
environment interpreted in one way or the other. There is,
further, a potential conflict between providing one sort of

'environment' or the other. Let us turn to this conflict first, because it provides the basis for a theme which recurs throughout this book.

A location for therapy (our first use of 'environment') derives its major characteristic from being an identifiable place; somewhere people go to receive therapy. In other words, its very separateness enables it to provide the facilities deemed necessary. Yet from the perspective of the setting as therapeutic (our second use of 'environment') it can be readily argued that settings which are separate, identifiable or distinct will not be so readily therapeutic. The argument here is essentially that in order to make people 'whole' or more like others in the community, it is essential to provide an environment which is part of the community and as similar to other normal environments as possible.

It can be seen, then, that revolving around a seemingly academic discussion of the meaning of the term 'therapeutic environment' can be a radical difference in administrative and design practice, say between providing a building complex with the latest facilities and aids on one hand, and modifying an existing building in the normal urban context which is not provided with much in the way of special facilities on the other, or indeed the extreme of providing community based services with no specific identifiable location; thus making the community a more therapeutic place to be, a place in which healing and caring is more likely to happen.

These are complex issues, yet they are significant for many aspects of daily life for many people within our society.

THE ROLE OF THE ENVIRONMENT

Symbolic qualities of the environment

The nature of the contribution of the physical surroundings to the therapeutic process can best be clarified with reference to two related roles which the physical surroundings can have. One is its symbolic role. The Victorian 'lunatic asylum' for example and its descendants, probably demonstrates more clearly than any other building form, with the possible exception of prisons, the attitudes which society has to the inmates and organisation which it houses. These large austere buildings, separated from the community, set in their parklands, epitomise the monolithic institutional processes which there have been so many pressures to reduce over recent years. It is an interesting thought that more benign building forms might have enabled these archaic organisations to linger on with less of a struggle than is now possible, because the buildings would not have demonstrated so clearly the need to do something about the institutions they house. Psychiatrists of a psycho-analytic frame of mind readily seize on these issues and Bettelheim, for example, has gone to great pains to elaborate a form of environment which he considers is symbolically appropriate for patients in writing about 'a home for the heart' (Bettelheim, 1974).

Indeed, the physical relationship which Freud himself espoused for the psycho-therapeutic interview in which the seated therapist is placed behind the encouched patient is taken, by cartoonists at least, as the symbolic epitomy of the psycho-analytic procedure. Exploration into the history of medicine and the activities, for example, of Mesmer also show the ready acceptance of the symbolic qualities of the physical surroundings, at the very least for setting the mood of the therapeutic interaction. It is even possible in Mesmer's case that these symbolic qualities were of greater significance than any other aspect of the process he utilised, and were certainly a more powerful explanation of the dramatic effects he produced than any reference to 'animal magnetism'.

Environments as facilitators

The symbolic qualities of the physical surroundings do derive, however, from the way in which those surroundings are playing their other role, namely, facilitating the therapeutic process. Whether a psycho-therapist places a desk between himself and his patient, a home for retarded children has sleeping accommodation near to a communally used kitchen, or an old people's home is placed close to a busy shopping centre, would all have an influence on the type of processes in which the participants of the setting may become involved. As discussed by Canter (1977), the fact that other people may 'read' from the physical setting the potential interactions which may take place and as a consequence elaborate from those interpretations ideas about, say, isolation or aloofness, which were not originally intended, helps to illustrate how seemingly small details may nonetheless grow to have great implications for symbolic interpretations. Hence 'institutional' colour schemes or imposing entrances may have an impact beyond their immediate function.

From the early work of contributors to this volume, such as Sommer, it has been apparent that details of the physical environment can have striking effects on socially related therapeutic processes. As Halohan demonstrates, the

type and arrangement of the furniture in a lounge area, for
example, can have a marked relationship with the pattern of
interactions which take place within the lounge. If social
discourse with others is considered an important part of a
therapeutic milieu, then the awareness that rows of cushioned
chairs are likely to yield high frequencies of detached unsocial behaviour, and that the reverse is true of light
chairs clustered around tables, may well be of some direct
clinical significance. Of even greater significance is the
role which the introduction of a change of furniture can play
in the hospital setting. This is illustrated well in the
contribution by Halohan to the present volume. It illustrates clearly that considering the physical environment
independently of the organisational structure of the institution can be most misleading.

THE EFFECT OF THE ORGANISATION

The need to take the organisational ideology and structure into account when considering the influence of the
physical environment on therapeutic processes, is a recurring
theme of this book. This theme does have another important
implication for the contribution which the physical surroundings may make to the therapeutic process. One important
difference between a person and an organisation is that the
latter has an extended spatial structure. Therefore, in
order to comprehend an organisation and take advantage of it,
it is necessary to understand how it is arranged in space.
A patient in any hospital requires some idea as to where
senior or junior nurses are likely to be found and the likelihood of a doctor being present on the ward itself. Furthermore, the patient is likely to gain some understanding of
his changing state through his changing experience of the
setting, whether it be the locations he is moved to or the
places he becomes able to seek out. Forming such a picture
of the spatial arrangement of the organisation, with which
interaction is necessary in order to obtain therapeutic
assistance, illustrates the fact that any difficulty in
forming such a picture may well lead to a greater reliance
on whom and what can be seen at a particular point in time,
or at the very least to the individual patient being placed
in a very dependent role. The patient who understands how
the organisation operates and where people can be found is
likely to have a greater potential for active search to find
help and care than one who can only wait in the hope that
such facilities will be brought to him.

The significance of the potential passivity, introduced
by the patient not being able to form an understanding of

the environmental correlates of the therapeutic organisation,
is exaggerated for most of the patients who need help by
virtue of what Lawton calls, in his contribution, their
environmental docility. For many reasons the people who are
the participants of therapeutic environments are likely to
be less able than any other individuals in the community, to
interpret and react to the often very subtle cues of relevance. Old people may be simply physically less able to move
around and thus form an understanding of how things work. A
number of investigators (notably Sommer, 1969) have demonstrated that psychotic patients find it particularly difficult
to use chairs and space generally in a socially acceptable
fashion. People who are less socially effective, or who are
less intellectually capable than the majority of the population, are likely to be more at risk in an institutional
setting than say the average office worker or school teacher
is in the institutional settings in which they normally work.

THE PAUCITY OF RESEARCH

These are general principles which take on a variety of
different significances depending on the particular setting.
It is partly because there is such a wide range of therapeutic
settings and such a wide variation in their scale and the
approach which they house that this book was felt to be
necessary. Nonetheless it is surprising that there is such
a paucity of information about the design of therapeutic
environments derived from effective research processes.
There are a great many accounts in the literature of the
experiences of various individuals in setting up such facilities and, of course, there are many government publications
which describe the physical layout and design to be achieved.
However, it is rare for these documents to provide substantive
evidence for the recommendations they are making or the
decisions which were made. It is almost as if in the need
to get on with doing something useful little resources are
available for evaluating and studying what is being done.
Furthermore, most of the research which has been carried out
tends to be carried out with captive populations which aren't
likely to complain too much. Thus, as in many other areas
of psychology, the most highly studied group are children.
In compiling this book we also found it difficult to obtain
information on small institutions. Again it would seem that
the people involved in these institutions have relatively
little spare capacity either to carry out research themselves
or to make facilities available for outside researchers. It
is large institutions under central government control which
are most likely to have been opened to research exploration.

This does mean that the present book is biased towards studies of institutions which many people would agree are not in the vanguard of therapeutic activities. And it does raise an important question for future research and policy as to how effective research activities can be instituted which will obtain information on smaller, decentralised organisations.

We should not under emphasise the practical difficulties of the type of research which has been carried out and which is being proposed. The administrative difficulties alone in setting up most, if not all, of the studies described in this book are difficult to believe unless they have actually been experienced. The researcher, like a patient, must gain an understanding of the organisation and how it is housed. He must then obtain permission from a wide range of people who have authority over the therapeutic processes. This will frequently include central government or at least regional authority groups as well as the hierarchies within the institution itself. There is a further problem which is of both a theoretical as well as a practical nature. A building cannot be examined unless the therapeutic goal and context itself is clearly specified. Yet many buildings develop as part of a complex process in which many and varied goals are intertwined. Canter (1972) showed for example that some of the design decisions underlying the building of a new children's hospital related more directly to the physical limitations determined by existing buildings, and the urgency necessitated by the discovery of structural failures in existing buildings than by clearly articulated therapeutic goals.

SPECIFYING THERAPEUTIC GOALS

Failure in the creation of therapeutic environments can frequently be traced to inadequate definition of therapeutic goals. It is not enough to set up objectives for therapeutic organisation as 'healing' or 'taking care' of people. Furthermore, describing the disabilities to be treated, whether of the blind, the mentally ill, the aged, the subnormal, or any other group, as produced by internal processes which need to be improved, frequently offers little in the way of specific guidelines for therapy. What is necessary is a way of specifying therapeutic aims which enables the setting to be considered as a direct facilitator of those aims.

Kushlick (1975) has gone to some considerable length to point out two of the confusions endemic in consideration of therapeutic environments. The first emphasises the ambiguous forms in which the goals of therapeutic settings are

established. The second relates to the wide range of individuals who work in therapeutic settings and the wide variety
of contacts which those individuals have with patients. He
elaborates the first problem of confusion in goal statements
by taking a lead from the work of Mager (1972). This leads
him to distinguish between what he calls a 'performance' and
a 'fuzzy'. To distinguish these from one another, Mager uses
the 'Hey Dad' test, for example:

"Hey Dad let me show how I can: increases this child's
attention; change his attitudes; improve hospital morale;
co-ordinate services."

These are called fuzzies because Dad cannot observe
whether or not I have done what I tell him that I have done.
A different set of Hey Dad items may be called performances
because Dad can observe whether or not I have done these
things.

"Hey Dad, let me show you how I can; set a goal for this
person; record what he did yesterday between 10.15 and 10.20
a.m.; arrange material for his learning to walk or dress;
graph the changes since last week."

Of course by forcing us away from what he calls fuzzies
towards performances Kushlick is taking a classical behaviour-
ist stand against what might be interpreted as a more humanitarian approach. However, there is little doubt that many
policy documents characteristically attempt to explain unobservable phenomena by the presence of other phenomena which are
also likely to be unobservable. In doing this it is frequently the case that a set of imponderables are set in motion
which make it particularly difficult for the policy maker, or
for the researcher to come up with any firm conclusions as
to the efficiency of the procedures proposed. Consider the
example which Kushlick gives, quoting from MacGillvary (1972)
giving an account of accommodation for the mentally defective:

"The mental state is, in the large majority of cases,
the result of illness, either genetically determined or the
result of pathological processes, which as a rule occur in
the interuterine state although a small number are caused by
severe brain damage post-natally."

Kushlick points out that in this statement which on the
face of it seems reasonably clear cut, a number of causes and
explanations are given which do in effect remove the possibility of considering the therapeutic setting directly and
lead to the continuation of the discussion in rather amorphous

terms. For example he points out that the term 'mental state' is used instead of behaviour, even though the term behaviour would not logically change the meaning of the statement, yet it would point to issues more directly available for scrutiny. Furthermore Kushlick points out that:

"The attribution of the cause of the client's day to day or minute to minute behaviour as 'genes' or pathological processes which cannot be altered, goes against the scientific evidence and the common sense proposition that minute to minute behaviour is controlled and can be altered by the way in which the environment responds to it."

In trying to establish clearly the goals which a therapeutic setting has, it is necessary to clarify many of the fuzzies which the policy makers may have established. This does not necessarily imply, as may be supposed from Kushlick's statements, that a strict reference solely to behaviour is essential. It may be necessary to put more reliance on verbal monitoring devices, such as those described in Sommer's contribution, or on records of what can be seen in an institution such as its level of cleanliness or the lockers which are provided, as illustrated in the contribution from Mazis and Canter. Or it may even be necessary to build up a detailed picture of the experiences of the individual and the way he relates to his setting as illustrated in the studies which Richer describes. All of these approaches are much more readily open to public scrutiny and therefore not so open to the whims and vagaries of the particular opinions of a particular management or policy making group. Nonetheless, the difficulty is still maintained that the organisation is talking and thinking in terms of fuzzies and the researcher is trying to deal in terms of clearly identifiable activities and experiences and thus the impact of research is less potent than it might otherwise be. This points to the way in which research can be of more value as an educational tool than as a policy guideline. It can often lead policy makers to formulate their ideas more clearly and thus open those ideas to more logical scrutiny with the consequent improvement in the service provided, even though substantive proposals from research may not be possible.

DIFFERENCES IN STAFF ROLES

The other complexity which Kushlick (1975) illustrates in detail is that the individuals who may interact with the clients in the therapeutic setting can be very varied and have very different roles. Frequently the discussions and decisions may be made by one group about the activities of another group. Yet the researcher may be in contact with a further, different group. Kushlick identifies four broad groups of individuals that may be found in a therapeutic setting.

"At the top of the list are the clients. Contacting and interacting directly with the clients are direct care staff. We distinguish:

I   The direct care twenty-four hours - these are members of the client's family (often a parent or spouse). The interactions with the client are likely to take place mainly in a single location every day of the week.

II   Direct care twelve hours - these include people like nurses, houseparents, assistants in residential settings who interact with clients mainly in the same location on a shift basis.

III Direct care two to six hours - include teachers, occupational therapists etc. who run programmes during a morning or afternoon of the five day working week. Their interactions with clients tend also to occur in the same location.

IV   Direct care ten minutes - this category includes people like doctors, social workers, educational/clinical psychologists, speech therapists, physiotherapists etc. They interact with clients in many different locations throughout the day; we call them the hit and runners and include ourselves, the researchers, among them. Very often, they interact mainly with direct care staff twenty-four hours, twelve hours or two to six hours who are the mediators between them and the clients.

Next come the monitors and supervisors. These include administrators and managers in social work, nursing, education, medicine, as well as professional managers or administrators. They tend to interact only with direct care staff and not with clients. They allocate resources between direct care staff working in different locations. They also monitor and supervise the way in which the direct care staff work.

Finally, there are the providers and planners. Their main interaction is with monitors and supervisors. They produce policy documents and circulars containing rules or guidelines to be followed or implemented by the monitors and supervisors. They also produce building notes (also rules) which predetermine the shape, size and components of facilities in which direct care activities will take place, i.e.

in which direct care staff and clients will interact throughout the day and night. Finally, they also provide the money
with which monitors and supervisors buy physical and personal
resources."

The problems of the institution as indicated by writers
such as Goffman (1961) and Tizard et al. (1972) can be traced
in part to the communication complexities inherent in the
organizational structure implied by Kushlick's categorization.
The generality of these organizational structures lead to
the fact that it is 'models' which most readily characterize
them and which may be transmitted through them. Any communication process is liable to give added weight and exag-
geration to the central themes which are being communicated
and those as complex as the ones found in a therapeutic
setting are liable to emphasize the themes underlying the
central assumptions about the facility. Given that so many
of the conceptions are essentially vague it is therefore
likely that the only real message on which agreement is
achieved can be characterized as a central stereotype or
model of the nature of the therapeutic situation. This idea
of a model, therefore, may be extremely helpful in enabling
us to identify the nature of an organization's approach to
any particular therapeutic setting.

The Custodial Model

To illustrate the idea of a model and its utility in
describing therapeutic environments we can begin with the
most obvious approach to providing facilities for those who
are considered to be different and less effective than those
in the rest of society. This model has certainly not dis-
appeared although it is probably the earliest articulated
perspective on provision of therapeutic facilities. Because
it has its clearest epitomization in the prison it is best
referred to as the 'custodial' model.

It will be remembered that a custodian is not necessarily a man of evil. In mythology he can certainly be a
protector of things of importance. As a consequence individuals in society who either needed to be protected from
themselves, from whom society needs to be protected, or who
indeed may need to be protected from the evils which society
may do unto them, have always been potential candidates for
being put under the care of a custodian. The essence of
the custodial situation is that individuals are separated
and protected from the community at large with a corollary
that the community at large is separated and protected from
them. Once it is agreed that for economies and efficiencies
of management it is necessary to put a number of these people
together in the same place then many of the initial custodial

goals may be negated. Indeed, as Sommer (1976) has pointed out, the early penal theorists felt that if prisoners were to be put together in a prison they must be kept separate in isolated cells so that they could not have a negative influence on each other.

Once individuals are brought together in groups, however, it is easy for the custodial model to degenerate into that of 'warehousing'. The individuals are kept together in one place, in effect stored in a reasonably non-debilitating environment, and an attempt is made to make sure that 'the goods', so to speak, cannot be stolen. There are clear indications that many of the long-stay facilities either for psychotic patients or for mentally retarded children have in the past been organised around the custodial, warehousing perspective. The contribution by the Gunzburgs is a clear attempt to move away from all the inhumanities which this perspective has left to posterity.

The Medical Model

In many ways the orientation which came in the 19th century with the great developments in medical technology can be seen as the first major inroad into the custodial model, replacing it with the 'medical model'. The changed perspective led to the view that all clients were, in effect, disease ridden, or 'unhealthy', and that as a consequence they needed to be kept in a setting where the appropriate medical treatment could be given to them so that they would regain their health. The power of surgical processes and of various forms of drugs, demonstrated in the area of general medicine that this orientation could achieve dramatic successes. Further, after Lister's introduction of antiseptics, it became apparent that many of the illnesses and diseases from which people had been suffering in hospitals were a product of the hospital setting itself. Florence Nightingale's often quoted statement "that at the very least hospitals should not make patients worse" was probably a direct reference to the effects of cross infection and the impact of poor hygiene on people undergoing treatment. As a result nursing procedures were based upon careful attention to hygiene and the appropriate distribution of medicines as well as the effective monitoring of the patient's state. There is little doubt that this approach has contributed in a large part to the change over the last hundred and fifty years in the experience of hospitals for patients. Indeed the change from going into hospital to die to going into hospital to recover is in no small measure due to the power of the medical orientation.

There does seem to be a tendency in human affairs for an approach which is found effective in one setting to be generalised to a wide range of other settings. There is, as a consequence, considerable evidence that the medical model has found its way into practically all other therapeutic settings. Many writers have explored the nature of this model, with its emphasis on the client as a patient who has an illness which is to be cured and the consequent emphasis on the individual's physical state, the general level of hygiene in which he lives and the further reduction in concern with the patient as a person. Richer's contribution shows the directions in which a medical approach to autism has led, for example, and Sommer and Kroll point out the inappropriate environments left in its wake. Furthermore, the contribution by Kenny and Canter shows that even within the acute hospital setting the power of the medical model may have influences which are counteractive to a truly therapeutic approach.

The Prosthetic Model

In attempts to get beyond the debilitating effects of dealing with participants in a therapeutic setting as 'patients', a variety of other perspectives have emerged in recent years. A range of variants of them will be found in the contributions to this volume. One of the most clearly articulated orientations which has been put forward as an attempt to get away from the idea of a patient who is to be healed is that which takes its analogy from prostheses. Kushlick (1975) gives the clearest definition of this:

"Prostheses compensate for deficits of behaviour or experience of an individual. For example, spectacles, walking sticks, bathrails, if used appropriately, provide compensation for certain lost or diminished skills. The individual is likely to be dependent upon such devices unless specific teaching methods are used gradually to enable him to do without them. This may not be important with such physical prostheses which may then become a permanent feature of the person's life. However, there are also social prostheses where, instead of a mechanical device another person is used to compensate for lost skills. Thus a 'home help' provides certain housework skills for an individual, 'meals on wheels' provide cooking skills. When an old person enters a home or hospital it is likely that many activities they previously performed will now be done for them by someone else. In some cases the admission to hospital may result in virtually all the patient's behaviour being socially prosthetised whereas dependence on physical prostheses may not be important, dependence on other individuals for a wide range of daily activity may be undesirable, particularly if at some time the people who do the supporting will be unable to carry on."

Whatever Kushlick's warning of the potential dangers of the prosthetic approach, it is clear that this approach has influenced the design of many therapeutic facilities. The most notable cases are those where physical prostheses are provided to enable people to cope with physical handicaps. Homes for the blind or for the physically disabled will frequently be considered in some detail from a prosthetic perspective in order that everything is done to enable the residents to work without the need for social prostheses. The obvious examples are handrails and ramps for people who have difficulty in moving upstairs, changes in textures for the blind or facilities at different heights for children. In our cities, in general, there is growing criticism of the lack of prosthetic devices to enable those whose physical abilities are not average. Anyone who suddenly finds that they have to move around their normal environment on crutches will quickly learn how more effectively prosthetic the environment could be and thus make their task much easier.

Nonetheless, Kushlick's warning can have significance for physically prosthetic environments as well as social ones. Wolff's contribution to the present volume points out how a 'non-prosthetic' play setting can have dramatic value for handicapped children.

Normalisation

As Kushlick warned and Wolff has demonstrated, then, the long term negative consequences of the provision of both physical and social prostheses may be great. If the individual comes to rely upon the crutch provided by the environment he may both become more dependent upon that crutch and less able to achieve whatever level of normal activity he can. As a consequence, a developing argument has emerged, which is most effectively argued in the contribution from Gunzburg and Gunzburg. They put forward the viewpoint that the therapeutic setting must be as normal as possible. This may well give rise to difficulties for the client initially. But it is argued that with appropriate training and help they can learn to overcome these difficulties and thus broaden the range of their possible activities and settings in which those activities can take place. Clearly, discussion of the appropriateness of the normalisation model will depend upon the severity of the abnormality of the client who is being considered. Nonetheless it shows something of the paradoxical difficulties inherent in thinking about therapeutic settings that it is necessary to articulate clearly what it means for a setting to be normal.

Usually normality is taken as more or less directly akin to 'domesticity' which is another frequent goal of policy makers. But the range and variety of domestic settings is doubtless so great that no single one can be held up for comparison with an institutional setting. Furthermore, there are certain logical inconsistencies in considering a setting which may house a large number of similar people with a few appointed senior people in charge, as in any sense parallel to a 'family'. Nonetheless many of the details of a family home can be shown to be essential to an effective therapeutic setting if it is to achieve the normalisation goal. It certainly undermines the implications of the medical model of cleanliness and the dependence on drug control of behaviour. Having facilities which can be owned and controlled by the individual as would be the case within a family are given much more emphasis in a 'normal environment' than would be the case in a medical environment where hygiene would be seen to be dominant. It is this view which makes Mazis and Canter's contribution so intriguing because it does indicate those aspects of the physical environment of institutions which help to contribute to their 'normalisation' and related client-centredness.

Enhancement

More recently an argument has been put forward that the 'normal' model is far too optimistic and ignores the fact that people in residential settings have great deficiencies for which allowances need to be made. In some ways this is rather similar to the prosthetic model where supports are provided within the environment. However, the approach which suggests that the environment must be enhanced, implicitly accepts that, by viture of being an institution, there is a potential for the setting being inevitably less rich than those settings available to non-institutional groups. As a consequence, attempts must be made to enhance the environment and thus counteract other aspects generated by the institution. The most detailed account of this approach is given by Sandu and Hendriks-Jansen (1976). They are concerned with severely handicapped children but their orientation implies a model which has more general applicability.

At the simplest level the enhancement model indicates that the physical surroundings should be livelier and more colourful than would normally be found, and thus counteract the drabness that is otherwise characteristic of institutional life. However it is argued that this enhancement of the physical setting should have some organisation and structure to it and thus make it much easier for the residents to understand both the arrangement of the spaces and of the organisation within space. In essence, taking Lawton's docility hypothesis as a very general statement of the difficulties people have in making sense of their physical surroundings, then the enhancement model suggests the task should be made as simple as possible for them by means of the design and layout of the facilities. This may be the bright colouring of walls and ceilings or it may go further towards the exploration of the possibilities of the type of facility described by Paul Wolff, whereby it is argued that handicapped children have even more need of the enhanced adventure playground type of facility than might the non-handicapped child.

The Individual Growth Model

The enhancement approach can be taken perhaps to its ultimate with the argument that the therapeutic facility is established to enable people to grow to their full potential despite the limited personal resources they might have available. Clearly such a model has implications beyond the physical surroundings. It implies many things about the contact between staff and patients and about the development of the staff/resident relationship over time. However, simply by virtue of the fact that development and change is anticipated there are implications about the changing processes which will make changing demands upon the physical setting. Thus although there may not be implications of a direct kind for the contents of the setting, there may be direct implications for its structure and organisation. Beyond the need for the environment to respond to developments and changes in general, the growth orientation also implies that each individual has idiosyncratic tendencies which must be nurtured. As a consequence, more than any of the other models, with the possible exception of the normalisation model, the growth model points to the need for involvement by staff and patients in the therapeutic setting and the opportunity for 'the personal touch' to find expression so that the growth potential for the particular individual is maximised.

Of course, by postulating the objective of enabling an individual to achieve his potential, the risk is run of specifying this objective in 'fuzzies' rather than 'performances'. By its very nature a person's <u>potential</u> is not at present available for objective scrutiny. This is all the more reason to emphasise the process, or procedures, which should be available in the setting, what the possibilities available to the client are. This returns us to the need to identify the symbolic qualities of the setting; what opportunities the client can see as available to him, and the facilities which he can actually draw upon. But using these possibilities depends upon what the organisational framework makes available.

THE SIGNIFICANCE OF EVALUATION

The journey from custodial institutions to settings for individual growth is a complex and arduous one. Along this journey a number of changes in emphasis are apparent and may serve to illustrate the general themes underlying subsequent discussions in this book. One is a change away from thinking of the total setting in the abstract to thinking of the details of the interaction between individuals in the setting. Related to this is a second theme of being less concerned for the goals and objectives of the organisation and more for the concerns and aspirations of the client. In physical terms the central implication of this is to change the direction of attention from a concern for grand, master plans and elegant design solutions towards a consideration of the actual materials and equipment over which the individual resident, patient, or client has control.

In the recent history of architecture there has been considerable discussion about the value of designing buildings from the inside out; making the external form reflect the internal requirements of particular spaces. This is always proposed as being in opposition to the school of thought which considers the production of the appropriate facade, or even of the most elegant plan form, being the essence of architecture. There are clearly parallels in the models discussed. Just as in architecture the tradition of producing the most effective facade still dominates the concern to obtain the most appropriate internal spaces, so in most therapeutic settings the desire to get the details of the facility appropriate for the particular client relationships is usually outweighed by the consideration of the broad strategies for keeping patients secure and clean.

It seems possible that details may be rendered ineffective if the general plan is inappropriate for those details. For example, no amount of attention to the location of particular pieces of furniture or the type of furniture which is provided in a particular room, with the consequent desire to modify furniture in relation to the uses made of rooms, can counteract a centralised ordering policy which sees dramatic economic benefits in ordering all furniture in the same style from the same manufacturer. On the other hand, it is the case that no amount of sophistication in making sure that the overall plan and administrative organisation is effective will ensure that particular details work. Details will only be effective if the individuals in the particular situations can have some influence over them. However, the need for central control and accountability does imply that some form of monitoring is necessary in the local situation. There does thus occur the implication that, provided institutional and therapeutic settings continue to be supported from public funds, increasing autonomy or attention to detail will require increasingly sophisticated monitoring procedures so that local abuses are not perpetuated. The evaluation procedures discussed by Kenny and Canter and those illustrated by Sommer and Kroll, Rivlin and Wolfe, and Mazis and Canter may thus be seen to have an increasingly important role in making therapeutic environments possible.

This book is concerned in the main with facilities which already exist. It is an exploration of what has been done in the past and an indication as to why it is that a new wave of approaches and facilities to therapeutic settings is emerging. In general then the value of this book will not be found in pointing clearly to specific, new, generalisable solutions. Indeed, our growing understanding of therapeutic process and therapeutic environments warns us against the search for general solutions. The value of this book therefore is to be sought in the clarification it provides of the different approaches which have been employed together with their advantages and disadvantages. Its most particular value is likely to be in highlighting current and past mistakes so that there is little excuse for them being repeated in the future. It seems to be one of the recurrent pitfalls of design that fashion gives way to fashion rather than more effective solutions evolving out of less effective ones. Effective evolution of design requires a careful consideration and evaluation of what has been achieved in the past. It is believed that by providing such an evaluation and clarification this book provides the goundwork for the radical improvement of our therapeutic environments.

SUMMARY OF CONTRIBUTIONS

The contributions have been placed in a sequence which approximately follows the provision of therapeutic facilities from childhood to old age. The first four papers deal with settings for children. The following two consider places which typically house young adults. Adult psychiatric facilities are then the focus of attention in a further two papers and are followed by two contributions dealing with geriatric facilities. A final contribution examines the evaluation of the acute general hospital as a therapeutic setting. The book is closed with an attempt by the editors to summarise the major directions for the design and management of therapeutic environments.

The sequence of contributions is intended to provide a reasonably direct route through the wide range of environments being considered. But the sequence also serves to illustrate how many of the developments in design and much of the research effort has related to a consideration of children. It may well be that the therapeutic goals here can be more clearly defined and also that the benefits of any environmental intervention are more immediately apparent than, say, with a geriatric population. However, it also seems likely that the child population, as in so many other areas of psychological exploration, provides a captive group. Nonetheless, whatever the reasons, it is clear that much of what has been learnt from looking at environments for children could usefully be extended to other situations.

Because of the pointers for other settings provided by looking at environments for children, the first contribution, by Rivlin and Wolfe sets the scene for much of what follows in the remainder of the book, highlighting many of the recurring issues. They represent the great majority of contributors who see therapeutic environments as a total community in a specific location. Over six years they adopted a multi-method, longitudinal approach to the study of the processes of adaptation and change of a centre specifically designed for emotionally disturbed children. In describing this centre they highlight a point which recurs in many later papers, that apart from therapeutic aims there is still the need to provide for normal experiences which the residents would have if not undergoing 'therapy'. With children this implies the provision for everyday socialisation processes and opportunities for freedom of choice rather than restricted control. With children it becomes apparent that the distinction between these 'normal' opportunities and 'therapy' is a difficult one to substantiate

and hence their paper implicitly raises the question as to
when such a distinction is tenable.

Rivlin and Wolfe demonstrate how both physical design
and management policy can create an institutional environment, even in a setting which by past standards is ostensibly
facilitative. Particularly striking is their description of
the differences between those involved in the planning, the
design and the running of the centre. It transpires that,
at times, the therapeutic aims of these three groups were
completely opposed. Moreover, none of the groups involved
in the production of this award winning centre, appear to
have given close attention to the way the building could
serve normal socialization processes, providing through such
factors as space, layout and furnishings a complement to a
treatment policy which would make available the opportunity
for the children to have those day-to-day experiences which
any child requires for its normal development.

The contribution by Richer which follows Rivlin and
Wolfe's provides a different view of the same central issues.
He considers four different settings for autistic children.
His sympathy is clearly with the use of those settings
generally inhabited by ordinary children of the same age as
autistic children, namely at home and school. Besides these
he examines an in-patient institution and a day care centre.
He expresses the view that future research should be concerned with finding the minimum deviations from those
provisions which are normally available which are essential
for adequate therapy. Like Rivlin and Wolfe, he also stresses the subtle interaction which takes place between the
physical and the organisational environment. Thus older
institutions frequently appear to lack the social organisation necessary to make best advantage of even the most
potentially creative physical settings.

Paul Wolff's paper emphasizes how much of what is of
value for one group of children can also be of value for
many others. The play facility he describes would be of
clear benefit to the great majority of children. His paper
gives an excellent review of the importance of creating a
suitable environment for both handicapped and other groups
of children. He reports a comparative study of the behaviour
of the same group of partially sighted children in a conventional and an adventure playground. The two play facilities
differed in both the physical provision and the administrative
structure. They show distinctly different patterns of social
behaviour. In one sense, the major discovery of his study
is that it is not the amount of physical activity which is

different in the two settings but the social quality of the behaviour which takes place. Wolff uses this finding to lend substance to his strongly argued support for the provision of adventure playgrounds for handicapped children.

Paul Wolff's contribution is the only one in this volume which deals directly with provision for the physically handicapped. One reason for this is that there are already excellent design recommendations available (e.g. Goldsmith, 1967, and publications by the London based Centre for Environment for the Handicapped). Another reason is that much of current thinking on design for the physically handicapped takes the approach that the places available to everybody else should also be made potentially available to those who, for various physical reasons, have in the past not been able to experience those locations. This approach is epitomised in the title of the Sheffield "Blind Mobility Research Unit" (e.g. James and Swain, 1975), whose goal is not to design special facilities for the blind, but to broaden their general mobility. They use a variety of training procedures and prosthetic devices, such as tactual maps. Perhaps, as Wolff reveals with adventure playgrounds, the end result of these explorations will be to make environments generally of value to all of us, not only to improve the design of therapeutic environments.

The last contribution to focus on environments for children is that by Mazis and Canter. They take up directly the theme of interaction between the organisation and physical provision referred to in earlier chapters measuring organisation and building in institutions for mentally retarded children. Their paper demonstrates the strong relationship between the measures of residential institutions derived from the work of King, Raynes and Tizard (1971) and physical details of those institutions. Their results show that a simple check list can be used to describe the design of a building. This list can then provide an index which has a high correlation with how child centred the organisation housed in the building is. The check list has the further value of providing a 'design tool' for generating building forms which will respond readily to child oriented management practice. The authors are, rightly, at pains to point out that no causal mechanism is implied by this strong correlation. Nonetheless, they clarify the important links which do exist between buildings and the organisations they house. In making these clarifications they point to some key physical correlates of child orientedness in a residential institution, notably the location of the kitchen, which finds an echo in the subsequent paper by Gunzburg and Gunzburg.

The Gunzburgs provide the unique combination of an architect and clinical psychologist who have been concerned for many years with creating appropriate environments for the mentally retarded of all ages. Their arguments are referred to by many contributors to this volume so it is appropriate to include a summary by them of the essence of their ideas. They argue for appropriate facilities to provide for three essential aspects for the development of the mentally retarded: socialisation, normalisation, and personalisation. They see the environment as contributing to the creation of learning opportunities for the residents by providing a setting which is essentially domestic in detail.

The paper following the Gunzburgs' shows some of the present limits on providing 'normal' environments for therapy. Sime and Sime describe a relatively unusual situation in which people convicted of various criminal offences are admitted to a unit run on psychiatric lines. It is debatable how confident the courts would be in sending people to a unit if it were not cast in a reasonably medical mould. Yet creating the appropriate environment is now a matter of very direct concern, ever since the report of the Butler Committee (1974) led to the recommendation that a 'medium security unit' should be provided in every health region in England.

Sime and Sime present the goals of the unit and in so doing illustrate some of the difficulties encountered with the 'fuzzies' discussed earlier. Yet through the detailed account of what happens in the unit it becomes clear that many of its goals are not achieved. The paper also serves to demonstrate how the building, designed originally for mentally retarded adults, contributes to the difficulty of achieving the organisation's therapeutic goals. The authors argue that in some ways the building has ossified a medical approach to its residents, with its wards, dayspaces, staff rooms and night station, which it is difficult for the current management to shake off.

Sommer and Kroll's paper serves as a timely reminder that there is still much to be done in evaluating and modifying what already exists if it is to reach present day standards of acceptability. Providing the background information for such modification is becoming an increasingly important research activity, not least in facilitating the renovation and improvement of existing state hospital buildings. However, Sommer and Kroll point out that if such contributions are to be of value they must be available shortly after the initial request to the researcher for assistance. The paper discusses the use of short question- naire surveys to answer this issue and presents the general conclusions of surveys conducted in two distinctly different psychiatric institutions.

As with other contributors Sommer and Kroll demonstrate that physical structure and social organisation interact in their effects, in particular that provisions for privacy can only be understood in relation to staff/patient ratios. They note the way in which the institution's requirements for supervision clash with patients' desire for privacy, especially in bathroom and toilet areas. They also support other studies which typically find that staff are more crit- ical of their environment than patients. This difference points to the difficulties of using questionnaire techniques in isolation of other methods, such as observation. None- theless, the authors point out that their perspective is frequently different to that of other specialists such as the engineer and that the survey itself can have direct value in raising the consciousness of the staff and in invol- ving the patients as people.

Following the hospital level of study of Sommer and Kroll's contribution, the second paper dealing with psychi- atric settings focuses on the spaces within a hospital. Halohan descrives two experiments, one dealing with the relationship between seating arrangements and social inter- action and the second with the remodelling of a traditional psychiatric ward. The significance of both these studies and the account given of them is that they are more than laboratory experiments which just happen to be carried out in the 'field'. They are explorations of the processes and effects of change within a psychiatric hospital. The relevance of this to the creation of therapeutic environments is that much of what is possible at the present time will involve introducing changes into existing settings. Halohan charts the processes of change. He argues that change in the physical environment is only likely to generate change in the behavioural and social system if the users of the setting are involved in the design. The resistance to change which they may otherwise express can negate the best inten- tioned designs.

Following the psychiatric facilities the contributions turn to considering provisions for the elderly. As the pro- portion of elderly people increases in society the provision of adequate housing and care facilities and appropriate environmental supports is becoming of major importance. Two papers provide substantial guidance for such provision, both in terms of what is to be achieved and how to achieve it.

Lawton provides an excellent review of the requirements for the elderly. He starts with a summary of what is known of the psychology of the aged, which is of relevance to environmental design. Considering the assets and disabilities of old people he discusses the provisions necessary to enable them to develop as individuals as well as to compensate for their deficiencies. He is able to show how an increased psychological understanding of the processes of aging has implications for many aspects of planning and design. It also becomes apparent, once again, as was clear when considering environments for children, that by making provisions for these 'abnormal' groups the environment will probably be more therapeutic for the rest of the community as well.

The second paper dealing with the aged, by Lipman and Slater, focuses more directly on the problem of the dependency of old people, which can so easily be exaggerated by the building and organisation created for their care. To deal with this they take the courageous step of proposing a design for a building which they believe will encourage more independence in its elderly residents through the provision of privacy, integration of various types of elderly and by the encouragement of personal and group activities amongst residents. The design proposed has a number of other more contentious implications which hopefully will stimulate deeper consideration of the planning and design of these increasingly important buildings.

The penultimate contribution, by Kenny and Canter, considers directly the design of acute general hospitals. It is surprising that the design of these buildings has, typically, been considered so separately from the design of the other therapeutic settings examined in this book. The reasons for this would be instructive to consider, but what is clear from the contribution by Kenny and Canter is that many of the problems and deficiencies apparent in these "non-medical" buildings are magnifications of those found in acute medical settings. This raises the possibility that much of what is wrong with the design of therapeutic environments is derived from the quintessential such location, the District General Hospital. However, before this argument can be taken further much more information is needed about user reactions to hospitals. Kenny and Canter review the existing literature and demonstrate that the processes of evaluation are a key to further understanding of hospital design. They highlight the complex organisation of the modern hospital and its built-in potential for diverse opinion about design. They further indicate that amongst such diversity of opinion it is frequently possible for the patients' reactions to be misinterpreted or forgotten.

The final paper is an attempt by the editors to indicate the major planning, design and management implications which are common to the papers in the book. These are presented as a set of questions which policy makers, designers or administrators should ask themselves about the places for which they are responsible. Answers are not spelled out in this presentation because they are so dependent on the particular context. However, many of the answers can be gleaned from the contributions to the book.

Finally, it is worth noting, that as long ago as 1957 Redl and Wineman, in discussing a facility for helping aggressive children, wrote of how they had found the need to create "a House that smiles, Props which invite, Space which allows" (p. 284). Nonetheless, it appears that only now are we beginning to build upon those early insights to a coherent understanding of what is the appropriate physical design for Therapeutic Environments. Many of the contributors to the present volume have followed their understanding through to design proposals, and in some cases to seeing their proposals built. For example, Lipman and Slater have given a detailed account of their proposed design solution. Wolff, Gunzburg, and Lawton have all seen their proposals through to actually being built. For the serious designer then, there are now places which can be visited to see what happens in practice. This book provides much of the ideas behind those places, but we have every reason to believe that it is part of a new approach to design in general, and therapeutic environments in particular. An approach which is based on an understanding of the organisational, social and psychological processes involved in the relationship between people and their surroundings.

REFERENCES

BETTELHEIM, B. (1974) A Home for the Heart, London: Thames and Hudson.

BUTLER COMMITTEE (1974) Report on Mentally Abnormal Offenders, London: HMSO (Command No. 5698)

CANTER, D. (1972) "Royal Hospital for Sick Children: A Psychological Analysis", Architect's Journal, 6th September, pp 525-564.

CANTER, D. (1977) The Psychology of Place, London: Architectural Press.

CUMMING, J. and CUMMING, E. (1964) Ego and Milieu: Theory and Practice of Environmental Therapy, London: Tavistock Publications.

GOFFMAN, E. (1961) Asylums: Essays on the Social Situations of Mental Patients and other Inmates, New York: Anchor.

GOLDSMITH, S. (1967) Designing for the Disabled: 2nd Ed., London: RIBA.

JAMES, G. and SWAIN, R. (1975) "Learning Bus Routes Using a Tactual Map", New Outlook for the Blind, pp. 212-217.

JONES, M. (1952) Social Psychiatry, London: Tavistock Publications.

JONES, M. (1962) Social Psychiatry in the Community, in Hospitals and in Prisons, Springfield IU: Chas. C. Thomas.

KING, R. D., RAYNES, N. W. and TIZARD, J. (1971) Patterns of Residential Care: Sociological Studies in Institutions for Handicapped Children, London: Routledge and Kegan Paul.

28

KUSHLICK, A. (1975) "Some Ways of Setting, Monitoring, and Attaining Objectives for Services for Disabled People", Winchester: Wessex Region Health Authority, Research Report No. 116.

MACGILLIVARY, R. C. (1972) "Accommodation for the Mentally Defective", Scottish Hospital Centre Conference (quoted in Kushlick, 1975).

REDL, F., and WINEMAN, D. (1957) The Aggressive Child, Glencoe, Illinois, Free Press.

SANDHU, J. S. and HENDRIKS-JANSEN, H. (1976) Environmental Design for Handicapped Children, Farnborough: Saxon House.

SOMMER, R. (1969) Personal Space: The Behavioural Basis of Design, Englewood Cliffs: Prentice Hall.

SOMMER, R. (1976) The End of Imprisonment, New York: Oxford University Press.

TIZARD, B., COOPERMAN, O., JOSEPH, A., and TIZARD, J. (1972) "Environmental Effects of Language Development", Child Development, 43.

Understanding and Evaluating Therapeutic Environments for Children

LEANNE RIVLIN AND MAXINE WOLFE

WHAT IS A THERAPEUTIC ENVIRONMENT?

The term 'therapeutic environment' may appear to have a clear meaning, yet even a superficial look at literature dealing with this area reveals a diversity of interpretations (Bettelheim, 1974; Trieschmen et al, 1969; Kugel and Wolfensberger, 1969). There is a real need to have a conception of therapeutic, a view of the areas of life that are encompassed and on the basis of this conceptualization, an understanding of culturally-defined therapeutic environments. Only then is it possible to consider whether environments defined as therapeutic actually serve their purposes.

Before presenting the conception of 'therapeutic' and 'environment' that is the perspective of our own work, it is important to look at the ways these terms are commonly applied. Usual definitions of 'therapeutic' focus on a specific group of persons who are identified as requiring treatment. They go by many different names, depending upon their cultural group's definition of their problem: emotionally disturbed, physically disabled, mentally retarded, elderly, sick, but they join in the common experience of being designated as different and singled out for a specific form of care. This isolation based on problem definitions has an environmental component as well. The physical isolation of the disabled in places specifically defined for special care enhances their stigmatization. The names of these places parallel the definition of the individual's perceived disability - psychiatric hospitals, homes for the aged and medical facilities. The combined social and physical designation of groups of people with a specific disability and a type of place to treat the disability has produced the modern structure we call an institution. The

29

type of therapy provided in these places closely follows
the rationale for defining the particular group. What is
generally emphasized is a curative or remedial process aimed
at either bringing the individual back into the mainstream
(as in the case of medical or psychiatric care) or at the
least, supporting the inadequate areas (as in the case of
the retarded, physically disabled or elderly). However, it
is not clear that settings so defined and delimited serve
a therapeutic goal. What is apparent is that by virtue of
their population, design and programming, they are recognized
as appropriate places for therapy.

The definition of problems and the explanation of their
etiology form the basis for the selection of experiences
and settings that presumably will lead the disabled back to
acceptable modes of behaviour. At this point in Western
society the system for categorizing problems is based on
two criteria: the ability of the person to take care of
themselves and the extent to which the person's behaviour
is perceived as a threat to themselves or others. Although
the physically handicapped, emotionally disturbed and mentally retarded have characteristics shared by everyone, by
these criteria they are separated out and labelled.

The perspective to be taken by the present authors is
one that places 'therapeutic' within the framework of general
development rather than extreme pathology. Acknowledging
that 'therapeutic' is a value laden term, in our view a
therapeutic environment is most simply one that recognizes
and supports both the strengths and weaknesses in people
(including physiological, psychological, social, economic
and political) without stigmatization and isolation. This
definition is intentionally broad in two respects - in terms
of the individuals involved and in terms of the conception
of environment. It emphasizes that while there are groups
of people who become defined and stigmatized as requiring
specific types of therapy, all of us need environmental
support to enable us to meet the requirements of our daily
lives and to grow and change over time. Our assumption is
that there are gross inadequacies in our ordinary living
environments which are a source of stress rather than support.
Studies of crowding, noise, transportation, and housing
attest to the limited attention paid to creating a humane
environment. This problem is even greater for individuals
with few options. By environmental support, we are referring
to a broad range of factors including physical, social, economic and political supports. The interdependence of these
factors in creating the settings in which we live means
that inadequacies in any one of these areas will affect the
others. For those with visual problems, one form of

environmental support is economic – the ability to obtain
proper diagnosis and treatment. The physical component in
the form of clear signs, proper lighting or large type in
newspapers can be an additional form of support. Political
influence can determine whether or not the particular disabled group can make its need known and implement change.
Any evaluation of the extent to which an 'environment' is
'therapeutic', therefore, requires studying a broad range
of people and environmental variables.

For a number of years we have been studying what has
been defined as a therapeutic environment for children with
emotional problems. The unique opportunity to enter the
facility prior to opening has resulted in a great deal of
information gathered over six years of occupancy. This
research has enabled us to gain a perspective on the changing
nature of all components in the complex system under study
and made it possible to understand what was happening on a
day-to-day basis in the lives of the people occupying this
setting. We began with the hypothesis that these systems
are open and dynamic. The research has supported this viewpoint and enabled us to understand the relationships among
changing conceptions of therapy, changing physical environments and the effects on all the people involved. We have
followed the evolution of this facility from a 'therapeutic'
into an 'institutional' environment.

THE SETTING FOR OUR RESEARCH

This children's facility, a low-rise building, was
awarded a prize for outstanding design supposedly providing
a contrast to the institutional-style architecture common
to most state facilities. It was designed to accommodate
192 children, ages 5 to 15. Providing total patient care,
the single structure included living areas, a school, therapy,
recreation and treatment facilities, in addition to administrative offices. The two-storey building rings an open
inner court, with eight foot wide corridors circling this
area and leading to other parts of the hospital (see Figure 1).
The experience of moving through the facility is one of
traversing long, maze-like corridors, despite the fact that
they are relieved in many places by glass panels and windows.
Eight 'houses' were designed to provide the living space,
with 24 children to be accommodated in each. They were
arranged in pairs, one above the other (one-half floor above
and one-half floor below the main level). The 48 children
in each set were to share a common dining room on the main
level, the food carted through a tunnel from the nearby
psychiatric hospital's kitchen (see Figure 2 for diagram of
the house areas).

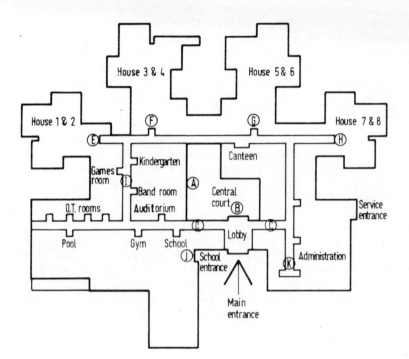

Figure 1: Floor plan

With the exception of two houses designed for autistic
children, the remaining six houses were identical in design.
A central corridor led to three living units or apartments,
each capable of accommodating eight children. Communal
areas for the three apartments consisted of a dayroom with
a kitchenette, a nurses' station, laundry room, office and
storage closets. Each living unit had a small entry foyer,
bathroom, living room and four bedrooms (two single rooms,
one two-bed room and a four-bed room). Two houses were
designed for autistic patients, and although their floor
space was identical to the other houses, only two rooms within each unit had walls, a large bedroom which was the sleeping and living area for the eight residents, and one two-bed
room.

Furnishings were selected by the architect and consisted
of beds with storage units and chairs and ottomans for living
rooms and dayrooms. An indoor-outdoor carpeting was used
to cover living unit floors. There was liberal use of glass
panels and large windows, both in the house areas and other
sectors.

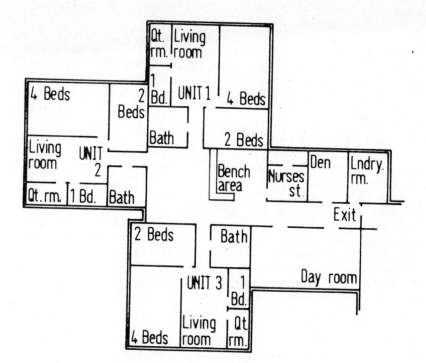

Figure 2: House 1 (Typical)

Community areas outside the houses in addition to a separate school wing, included a game room with pool tables and table tennis, a kindergarten room, music room, four occupational therapy rooms, a fully equipped gymnasium, a full-sized swimming pool, a library, auditorium and canteen. Each set of houses had an outdoor play area immediately behind, and the kindergarten room had direct access to its own play area in the centre court.

Methods

Our study has relied on a longitudinal methodology. The opportunity to be involved in one setting over a long period of time, gave us the advantage of being able to understand any particular change as part of an ongoing process. These data clarified the role that each component of the system contributed and militated against a simplistic architectural or social determinism. Based on this theoretical-methodological orientation, our research strategy has been to use a variety of methods: historical analysis, interviews with all the persons in the system, systematic observations focusing on both aggregate and individuals and studies of naturally occurring and planned changes.

Before the facility was opened, we reviewed the state programme and interviewed the architect and the newly appointed director. Beginning with the first day of occupancy, we visited bi-weekly, if not more often, and have systematically collected field notes indicating a variety of details including policy decisions, programme changes, and physical changes. We attended meetings at all levels of staff. We conducted seven systematic time sampling observation studies of the patterns of space use in the entire facility (living and community areas), the first in March 1970, the last in January 1976. We conducted an observational and interview study before and after the installation of bedroom doors; a study of children's cognitive maps of the facility, and an interview study of children's and staff's concepts of privacy, and a longitudinal tracking study following four children each for an entire day. We have used data from several studies to evaluate the use of bedrooms varying in amount of space and number of occupants and used data from nursing logs to evaluate the use of space as a control mechanism. We also helped the children and staff plan, design and implement the change of two seclusion rooms into den-type rooms, evaluating the effect of the changes through a pre-post time sampling and event sampling observational and interview study. Finally, the unplanned move of the adolescent girls to a living space with dormitory style sleeping arrangements following a fire in their living unit, formed the basis for a comparative observational and interview study.

This multi-method longitudinal approach has enabled us to use behavioural and attitudinal data as criteria against which to evaluate the various conceptions of 'therapeutic' which contributed to the facility's design and functioning, including: (1) the State Department of Mental Hygiene who developed the programme for the facility, (2) the architect who translated this programme into a physical form, (3) the director who implemented a treatment programme in this facility, (4) the staff, who on a day-to-day basis, carried out and redefined the therapeutic programme and (5) the children whose behaviours, feelings, attitudes and perceptions reflected and affected the therapeutic orientation, and finally, (6) the researchers' own conceptions which emerged out of prior experiences, as well as participation in this study.

Multiple conceptions of this therapeutic environment

In order to get a perspective on the variety of definitions of therapeutic that contributed to the concrete structure of the children's psychiatric hospital, we traced the
State Program written in 1964. The programme was merely a
series of space allocations for different types of services
and functions. Implicitly, however, the types, distributions
and allocations of spaces clearly reflected a medical model
of therapy. This was to be a residential facility providing
for all of the daily life experiences that the children
might need including school, recreational facilities, living
areas and a fully-equipped infirmary. The complete coverage
of every aspect of life implied that the total child needed
support. The site location of the hospital, a vast tract
of land shared by a series of other institutions, separated
from the surrounding community by highways and railroad yards,
implied that isolation from and protection of the community
was paramount. The elimination of doors on bathrooms and
bedrooms, a requirement of the Program, the constraint that
all services be located within one building, made control a
paramount part of the philosophy.

In his attempt to translate this programme into its
physical form, the architect added his own conceptions of
therapeutic, and attempted to modify what he perceived to
be the State's position. The scale of the physical form
which would be created by placing all services within one
building was at variance with the conceptions of therapeutic
that the architect found to be common in other children's
facilities considered to be of high quality. His modifications reflected an attempt to articulate and bound small
living areas on the scale of apartments, breaking up the
space to reduce the massive nature of a single buildings,
using materials and decoration that he felt would reduce
the institutional quality (glass, wood, carpeting, individual
bed and storage units). He wanted to provide for a wide
range of ordinary living experiences, which he believed could
evolve spontaneously if variations in scale were present.
There were many unchangeable conditions which he considered
to be an impediment to his goals - among them the number of
children to be housed, the width of corridors, the materials
used for demarcating spaces and the particular services to
be included.

The director was appointed after the building had been
completed and, therefore, had no input into the planning.
His philosophy of treatment was markedly at variance with
the original State Program. Although the director shared
many of the architect's values, he was not entirely

sympathetic to the form of the building. He believed that
he could achieve his goals within this physical form through
programming, politics and the exercise of a point of view.
He was a strong proponent of community based care. Although
no provisions for day care were included in the building, he
set an admissions policy of at least half day care patients.
Despite the inclusion of all services in the building, he
opened the facility to people in the community, inviting
them in. He also wanted wide use of community facilities
by the patients. He had no intention of using the infirmary,
believing that a mild illness should be treated in the residences (as it would at home) and serious ones in a regular
hospital. He planned to institute a series of different
programmes such as a tutorial, half day for children who
were not part of the hospital's population. Politically,
he intended to reduce the ascribed capacity of 192, and
eventually had it lowered to 125. In terms of a point of
view, he believed children should not be controlled by locked
doors, that they should have choices rather than be confined
to an inflexible institutional schedule. Trips, allowances
and highly individualized programmes, he felt would offset
the impact of the physical form. There were also some physical changes that he felt were essential; in particular,
installation of doors on toilets and bedrooms.

The researchers considered the three points of view
from the perspective of their own past experiences and phil-
osophic orientation. It was our hypothesis that the site
location would interfere with achieving the director's goal
of community interaction. Transportation both out to the
community and into the hospital area seemed to be a major
stumbling block. The isolation of the children's hospital
and its location next to a series of large adult psychiatric
buildings cast an even more intense symbolic separation from
the surrounding area. Despite an exterior design which was
unlike most institutional buidings, several other physical
qualities contradicted this impression. The landscaping
and provision of barbecue pits, basketball courts and baseball fields presented amenities but in a context that was
open and rather bleak. The scale of the building, the need
for a complex corridor system, symmetrically laid out and
physically identical living areas, the monotony of the materials which did not convey any obvious differentiation in
function, the lack of soft materials, the absence of internal
indications that children of different ages would be accommodated - all were components of other institutional settings,
although in a newer and more modern aesthetic. Two specific
aspects of the design that looked like potential problems
were the multiple occupancy bedrooms and lack of doors on
bedrooms and toilets. Both of these seemed to limit the

possibilities for privacy. In summary, it was clear that
the setting was in no way 'normalized' except at an abstract
level of conceptualization. It was hard to imagine that the
children who would live there would have ordinary experiences
of daily living.

FINDINGS AND IMPLICATIONS

Table 1 presents an overview summary of the major questions we studied. For each of a series of physical elements
within the hospital, we have indicated the implicit and
explicit assumptions of the State Program, the architect
and the director, and we have documented physical and administrative changes which occurred as well as data on actual
use and attitudes. A review of the table brings out certain
themes which are important in contrasting institutional and
therapeutic environments. This discussion will focus on
these themes using data where appropriate, although we will
not review all of the studies in depth (see references).

One theme which emerges is the strong influence of the
so-called 'therapeutic environment' as an institutional
socialization agent. The presence of the children in the
hospital is the end product of a labelling and segregating
process which calls for a specific type of socialization -
therapy. The lack of differentiation between these two
processes results in the institutionalization of children.
How is this done? As one example, the intense focus on the
problem aspects of these children created a social/physical
environment devoid of opportunities for most forms of privacy
available to children living in ordinary home environments.
The supposed need for surveillance and the goals of fostering
social interaction took precedence over general developmental
needs. Children spent most of their days in the presence
of others, were always accompanied, could not control access
to their bedrooms, and information about them was readily
available to all staff and other children. Being alone and
not sharing feelings or thoughts were interpreted as signs
of pathology rather than ordinary human needs. Our data on
concepts of privacy indicate that the hospitalized children
associated privacy with an extremely limited range of mean-
ings when compared to a matched sample of non-hospitalized
children. Notably absent were any elements of choice (doing
what you want to do), control over intrusion (no one bother-
ing me), control over access to spaces (no one can come in),
control over access to information (no one knows) and freedom
of movement. All of these aspects were mentioned by the
non-hospitalized groups. For hospitalized children, the
seclusion room was viewed ambivalently. It was the only

Table 1: Comparison of assumptions regarding use with actual
use over six years of children's hospital functioning

PHYSICAL ELEMENT	IMPLICIT ASSUMPTIONS	EXPLICIT ASSUMPTIONS
Capacity - 192	S: Economically viable for residential treatment.	S: Expected need. A: Too large. D: Too large; would never reach this level.
Site location	S: Children must be isolated from community - help patients; protect community; economically viable.	S: Land available. D: Maximum community contact needed.
Outdoor recreation	S: Recreation is therapeutic but should not use community facilities.	S: Provide total outdoor recreational needs. A: Provide age-designated outdoor facilities each connected to a specific house. Range and type of equipment varied. Mudrooms provide easy access.
4 separate but interconnected areas	A: Illusion = reality of separateness.	A: Would seem more like a normal environment.

A = Architect
S = State Department of Mental Hygiene
D = Director

CHANGES DURING OCCUPANCY (1970-1976)	DATA COLLECTED	FINDINGS ON USE (1970-1976)
D: Reduction to 125	L	Average day + full care = 60. Full care, maximum 35.
	L O	Major summertime use of community facilities; little community use of facility.
Area designed for youngest age group enclosed by wall. Softer materials substituted on swings.	O	Age related areas not used by age groups nor were age groups housed in adjacent areas. Adolescent seating area unused. Traditional playground used rarely in winter and fall, occasionally in spring and summer. Mudrooms did not provide expected access.
	O L	Administrative areas barred to children, leading to supervised travel.

L = logged
O = observations
I = interviews

PHYSICAL ELEMENT	IMPLICIT ASSUMPTIONS	EXPLICIT ASSUMPTIONS
Separate administrative wing 6,050 sq. ft.	S: Some administration shared with adjoining adult facility.	S: Administrative space sufficient. D: Administration not to be shared.
Diagnostic and treatment (physician's office, nurse's office, examining and treatment, EEG lab, dental treatment) 1,015 sq. ft.	S: Need separate services; more efficient.	
Infirmary - fully equipped - 2,695 sq. ft.	S: Children cannot use ordinary medical facilities. D: Children need normal community connections and experiences	S: Children require complete medical facility. D: Minor ailments should be treated in houses. If illness requires hospitalization, use community facilities.
School - 11,725 sq. ft.	S: Children need separate school facilities.	
4 O.T. Rooms	S: Various arts and crafts are therapeutic.	S: 4 rooms adequate. A: Sinks etc. make functional.

CHANGES DURING OCCUPANCY (1970-1976)	DATA COLLECTED	FINDINGS ON USE (1970-1976)
Immediately converted one house for additional administrative space and infirmary.	I	Never shared administration with adult hospital. Space always additional acquisition. Lack of therapy rooms.
Converted to administrative area and half-day tutorial programme.	O	Never used as intended.
After 1½ years, 4 O.T. rooms found inadequate; unused house converted to arts & crafts unit.	O	Therapists immediately found rooms too small and isolated. Initially used canteen as auxiliary space; then converted one house. Staff preferred this despite inadequate facilities.

PHYSICAL ELEMENT	IMPLICIT ASSUMPTIONS	EXPLICIT ASSUMPTIONS
Gym Pool Auditorium (seating 250)	S: Require separate facilities. A: Children given choice. D: Community will receive children in local facilities, programming can handle this.	S: Facilities appropriate. A: Many choices offered. D: Children should use facilities in surrounding community - not be isolated during treatment. Community people should use hospital facilities.
No daypatient	S: Residential	S: Children require total residential care D: Wanted outpatients to be 2½ times the number of inpatients.
Separate autistic wards		S: Autistic children require more surveillance because they are self-destructive and fear being alone. A: Design consistent with available literature. D: No sound basis for design. Grows from need to supervise and control rather than therapy.
Articulated houses	A: The illusion of separate houses = the reality of separate houses.	A: First choice - separate cottages to create more normal environment. Final design created illusion of individual houses placed in separate wings of building. D: Felt mirror-image house would confuse children with orientation problems. Disliked numerous corridors this design required.

CHANGES DURING OCCUPANCY (1970-1976)	DATA COLLECTED	FINDINGS ON USE (1970-1976)
	O	Community never used facilities. Pool rarely used until 3 years after opening; now used at programmed times. Full-sized gym rarely used by more than 10 children; unoccupied for large parts of day. Auditorium usually empty, sometimes used for movies or conferences.
From beginning, about half were day patients.		Daypatients had no space other than school; number decreased.
Never used as residential space for autistic children. One unit converted into OT spaces; doors built to separate spaces. Other unit used as offices and one living area used as day programme space for autistic children. After fire one unit used as temporary living space.	O	Never used as intended.
	O	Location of houses away from but connected by corridors to community area led to use for isolation and detention. Institutional structure did not allow use as actual apartment or houses. There were no problems in orientation perhaps because only 3 of 8 houses actually used as living spaces. Other houses renovated to serve other functions.

PHYSICAL ELEMENT	IMPLICIT ASSUMPTIONS	EXPLICIT ASSUMPTIONS
1, 2, 4 bedrooms	S: Bedroom size may not matter.	S: Since ages unknown provides needed flexibility. A: Initial choice: no demarcated bedrooms, furniture to partition area. Rejected by State. Second choice: an office-type partition Rejected by State. Final design of 1, 2, 4 areas would provide flexibility but not be optimal for any age. D: Single room preferable for all ages. Privacy needed and best achieved in own room. Felt 4-bed room would be problem - little available floor space.
No doors on bedrooms or bathrooms	S: Children need constant surveillance. D: Doors provide privacy for children.	A: (see bedrooms) D: Doors essential, exclusion stresses control.
Diversity of spaces in houses	1) Provision of diverse space will result in diverse use. 2) Analogy of home = home.	A: Each unit would be a small apartment with privacy and small group activities much as in a family setting. Communal space for large groups. Kitchenette would offset institutional food system.

NGES DURING UPANCY 70-1976)	DATA COLLECTED	FINDINGS ON USE (1970-1976)
	O I	Potential density not related to behaviour. Room size and group size interacted to create certain psychological density conditions. Private rooms used most often for behaviour for which no other space available. As number of children assigned to room increased, use of the room by each child decreased and interactive behaviours decreased. Two child bedrooms need more space than double that of one child room.
rs put up ut 5 years er opening.	O I	Privacy concepts of children strongly reflected their institutional experiences. Doors only closed 2% of the time. Initially a change in activity in bedrooms. 1½ years later original patterns found.
sed on past search, an vironmental tervention anned with tient part- ipation con- rted old iet room to den-type ace with ft furniture, ll panels, rpeting. tended as ace for ivacy.	O I	1) Regardless of differentiated size of interior house spaces, predominant behaviours were isolated. 2) Age differences were found in use of identical house areas. Adolescents were able to specify function and use similar spaces in differentiated fashion. Children's behaviours were similar regardless of room or ascribed function. 3) Dayroom never functions as spontaneous group meeting place; kitchenette rarely used. Dayroom functioned mainly to gather children for surveillance under low staff conditions. 4) Living rooms in living units (for 8 children) lowest use of all house areas. 5) "New room" used as planned - self-selected and non-punitive place for patients to be alone or be with one other person. Staff and children positively evaluated it especially for humaness of scale and truly non-institutional furnishings (see Amenities).

PHYSICAL ELEMENT	IMPLICIT ASSUMPTIONS	EXPLICIT ASSUMPTIONS
Amenities - carpeting, draperies, glass, low-hanging fixtures, personalized furniture.	A: These elements create non-institutional appearance.	A: A technique for de-institutionalizing the facility. Compromise between making it destructible, like a jungle or jail, and making it home-like. Poor maintenance would undermine. D: Lighting would become natural target for children - would have to be replaced. Non-institutional looking, but maintenance might be a problem.
No seclusion - quiet rooms	S: Attempt to avoid overt, punitive areas considered to be inhumane for children.	
Total amount of space - 80,885 sq. ft. (includes 10,685 sq. ft. for service areas)	S: This was amount necessary for all services for residential treatment.	

HANGES DURING CCUPANCY 1970-1976)	DATA COLLECTED	FINDINGS ON USE (1970-1976)
emoval of car- eting; removal f low-hanging ights; repla- ement of glass ith plexi- lass.	O I	1) In early stages, generally poor maintenance - general state of dis- repair led to elimination of carpet- ing, etc. Repetition of similar hard furniture worked against personaliza- tion and gave institutional feeling. 2) In "New Room" children took over maintenance and room has remained in good condition.
ffice in each ouse converted o quiet room. n all living nits used as on-residential paces, all imilar offices onverted into uiet rooms. ater, one ingle bedroom n each living nit converted o quiet room.	O I	As number of quiet rooms increased, the use of them increased. Intention to have staff person in room with child rarely occurred; children con- fined there alone when "disruptive".
	O	Space has always been too large for children and number of staff. Vast areas unused most of day and evening. One house now used as temporary space for group of developmentally disabled children; one house used temporarily for ½ day tutoring programme. One house partially used for day care autistic children.

PHYSICAL ELEMENT	IMPLICIT ASSUMPTIONS	EXPLICIT ASSUMPTIONS
Communal spaces (court, canteen, corridors)	A: Internal corridor can function as a street. Centre court and canteen would be used spontaneously and provide places for social interaction.	A: Would be used as spontaneous and programmed social interaction spaces. Re: corridor: original choice 12' with lounges providing "Main Street" effect. Now saw it as labyrinth. D: Vast, expansive corridor system would create problems for children with orientatio difficulties.
Murals, sculpted figures in court, etchings on walls (indoor and outside)	A: Children would be free to wander and enjoy these.	A: Provide an aesthetically pleasing and serendipidous experience in viewing/using them.

ANGES DURING CUPANCY 970-1976)	DATA COLLECTED	FINDINGS ON USE (1970-1976)
cess doors to urt, canteen and rridors kept cked.	0	1) Orientation problems did not materialize. 2) Corridors originally used for roller skating etc. Over time restricted to staff accompanied traffic and only used as transit from one programmed activity to another. Despite increases in number of occupants, the number of people in corridor decreased giving a sense of a deserted town. 3) Of several thousand activities observed in community areas, only 50-100 were observed in court and canteen. 4) Canteen not used until almost 3 years after opening. First used as auxiliary crafts area; then pool and ping pong tables moved in and used at programmed times as game room. Now used 3 or 4 times a year for occasional parties - accounts for 3.2% of all hospital activity.
er time, murals oliferated as t.side groups coraded cordors and houses.	0	1) Lack of interest in this perceived as institutional. 2) Murals described as "hospital art". 3) Sculptures never used as play objects.

PHYSICAL ELEMENT	IMPLICIT ASSUMPTIONS	EXPLICIT ASSUMPTIONS
Kindergarten Room and Play Area	A: Kindergarten-age children need easy access outdoors.	A: Need to segregate younger children in age-appropriate spaces. D: Design contained facilities (sinks, toilets, play area) to maxamize use.

ANGES DURING CUPANCY 970-1976)	DATA COLLECTED	FINDINGS ON USE (1970-1976)
ter one year con-rted to staff lib-ry. Youngest chil-en first placed in w arts and crafts use, access to tdoors created by ilding a staircase om a window to tdoor play area. is play area re-signed - fence nstructed, soft ings replace metal ings. After 6 nths, moved to a use used mainly r administration. outdoor play ea immediately cessible.	O	1) Used as intended for only one year. 2) Converted to staff library, thus equipment not rel-evant. 3) Frequently unused for months. 4) Outdoor play area "went to weeds".

acceptable place for uninterrupted solitariness but was also experienced as "the most uncomfortable place in the hospital". Children had to "act-out" in order to be sent there and, thus, aloneness became associated with emotional upset.

The major focus of the hospitalized children and staff was on "privacy for undressing and toileting" - a function so obvious in ordinary life that the non-hospitalized children hardly mentioned it. By focusing on this narrow but obvious issue, the manner in which the lack of other forms of privacy created an institutional and non-normalized socialization environment was totally overlooked. When one speculates about the possible effects of this narrow conception on the total life of children, it becomes apparent that limited preparation is provided for life beyond walls of this type of environment. For example, because of the association between aloneness and emotional upset, these children may have great difficulty dealing with the aloneness that is part of ordinary daily life. Goffman (1962) demonstrated the effect of such re-socialization on adults; we believe it is even more significant in the lives of children when institutional life provides the <u>primary</u> socialization experience.

The socialization impact of the institutional quality of this type of environment is further illustrated by our data on patterns of space use and behaviour. For a brief time early in the hospital's history, with limited staff and a small number of children, the facility was used in an unstructured and spontaneous manner. We saw roller skating in the corridors, doors were unlocked, children would request and be allowed to use various rooms, crisis intervention was the major therapeutic tool. Over time, the day became more structured and programmed, doors were locked, free travel restricted. The living units, physically isolated but accessible from community areas, became crystallized as areas of detention - a place to send children when "acting-out". Detention became even more localized as seclusion rooms were created within each living unit six months after occupancy. High energy behaviour was replaced by more passive and low energy activity. A stable pattern of behaviour evolved in the entire facility as well as in specific spaces, one that continued despite changes in children and staff.

It is also possible to view the impact of multiple bedroom types, ostensibly provided for flexibility, in light of the socializing impact on the children. Although this arrangement may have seemed to imply options for the administration, it is clear that certain bedroom types provided limited options for the children. Our data and that of others (Holahan and Saegert, 1973; Ittelson, Proshansky and Rivlin, 1970) combine with the literature on density (e.g. Hutt and Vaizey, 1966) to indicate that both the size of a space and the numbers who occupy it strongly affect the kinds of behaviours that occur. In a therapeutic context where children spend most of their days in programmed activities in the presence of other children, the options provided by various types of bedrooms must be viewed against the daily experiences possible given the varieties of available spaces.

In this facility, as in others, solitary behaviour was viewed as inappropriate in all but bedroom spaces. Our data showed that the amount of space and number of people in multiple occupancy rooms made it difficult for children to use these rooms for such behaviour. As a result, it was only the children in single-bed rooms for whom this was a viable option. Two-person bedrooms showed the least amount of use. Because of what seemed to be problems of the emotional dependency created in two-person spaces and the privacy problems, children in these rooms engaged in behaviours which could be interrupted (for example, housekeeping, hair combing). This seemed to be a clear example of how children can be socialized to the use of space even though their needs may not be met in the process.

A second theme is the extent to which so-called bureaucratic efficiency needs take precedence over therapeutic needs, either without awareness or with the belief that other procedures or experiences can be compensatory. This manifests itself in a variety of ways. For example, while all of those involved in the planning believed that eating and food preparation were central parts of a child's life and important normalizing and therapeutic activities, these goals were concretized only by the provision of a kitchenette in the houses. The kitchenettes were supposed to be used for spontaneous snacking. The three main meals were part of the programmed day, prepared in the adjacent adult hospital and served cafeteria-style in a separate dining room accommodating 48 children. Food preparation and serving was, therefore, seen as more economical (food was ordered in bulk for both the adult and children's facilities; equipment and staff did not have to be duplicated). Yet, because the dining room was not part of the house areas, eating required one more experience of 'lining up' and supervised travel. The physical separation, the use of a separate food serving staff who were not otherwise part of the children's daily life, the experience of eating with a large group of other children, all resulted in a strictly time-limited institutional eating experience. The house kitchenette was used mainly to store utensils for night-time snacks which were also prepared outside of the house areas. The belief that the inclusion of the kitchenette would offset the institutional food arrangements was based on the premise that its physical presence would creat use. Since the major nourishment was taken care of in the dining room and all preparation in the main facility, the kitchenette became nutritionally redundant, literally and figuratively non-functional and clearly uneconomical.

A third theme is the <u>inadequacy of "illusion equals reality" as a basis for design and programming</u>. Very often, the creation of physical/social environments which give only the illustion of normalcy is based on a perception of the need for a more human environment but the unwillingness to give up deeply ingrained notions of 'sickness' and 'treatment'. In a sense it represents an approach to change which often negates the possibility that change will occur. In this setting, the articulation of four separate but corridor-connected areas within a single building was supposed to be an analogy to the separation of these activities (school, living, recreational, specialized care) in ordinary life while still maintaining a reasonable degree of control over children's movements. However, the overall size of the building and the general notion that all activities were part of a 'therapeutic' life, led to the lack of free, un-accompanied movement from place to place and the strict programming for use of the areas. These areas became psychologically as well as physically connected. The use of any part of the facility was within the context of it as a single therapeutic entity and in no way paralleled the actual separation of these types of activities in the ordinary lives of children.

The physical articulation of separate houses, again, did not mean that they either were perceived of or functioned as usual living areas or apartments. In ordinary life, for example, the school is physically separate and at some distance from the home. This means that behavioural problems occurring in school are dealt with in school. Children are not sent home. In addition, the ordinary separation also gives children, at least above the age of eight, the opportunity to travel to and from school and to have the experience of time away from authority figures and time with or without peers depending on their choices. The use of an internal corridor system to connect the living areas to the rest of the facility meant that both of these experiences were negated. The houses were close enough to be used as areas of detention, requiring little effort to do so. Yet, the corridor system was long enough and went through enough

"off-limits" areas so that free movement was not permitted.
Children were always accompanied by staff. The houses may
have been visually separate but were not programmatically
or psychologically separate.

The attempt to make the houses seem home-like was
another example of the deception of analogies. The apartments or living units within these houses never functioned
as intended. The image cast by their being embedded in the
context of a glass-walled nursing station, a seclusion room
and a large dayroom, all behind the locked door leading to
the house areas, negated the supposed home-like qualities
of the smaller apartment units. While the living units had
several bedrooms and a living room, these were not readily
available to patients. The inability of nursing staff to
easily surveil the apartments from the nursing units meant
that they tended to herd the children into the dayroom or
corridor.

The materials used in these areas were no different
than those in the other hospital areas - white concrete
block walls, hard surfaces, tweedy, dark-coloured fabrics,
heavy wooden frames on chairs and sofas to ensure their
immobility. The furniture in the dayrooms and living rooms
was the same as that in the canteen - a community space as
opposed to a home space. Despite the provision of so-called
home-like amenities, their effect was negated by design,
physical details, and attitudes that were institutional in
quality. Missing throughout the entire period of our study
were indications of personalization of spaces or evidence
of daily human living. Nothing was out of place; no small
objects were visible on table tops. Anything affixed to the
concrete walls fell off, resulting in the use of painted
graphics to fill up empty wall space. When we worked with
the children to renovate two seclusion rooms into den-type
spaces, the result of their choices was a room with wood
panelling, soft furniture with bright red fabric, pink walls
and a red carpet. The children and staff alike described
it as the most "home-like" place in the hospital commenting
especially on its softness and coziness. During the planning
process one staff member suggested graphics for the wall.
The overwhelming response of the children was negative -
"you don't have designs painted on the walls at home".

To some extent the use of such illusions are based on
the perception that these children will not be sensitive to
the substitution of an analogy for the real thing. Our
experience shows that this is just not true and, in fact,
the children are very aware of the extent to which these

are just illusions. One can question the therapeutic value
of the conflicting messages given to the children by the
use of such illusions.

A fourth theme is that access is not simply a function
of the presence of physical elements or the functional designation of spaces. On paper, this facility, as well as
others, seem to have an impressive array of environmental
possibilities - gymnasium, canteen, arts and crafts, pool,
outdoor recreational areas - and many means of access -
doors, glass panelling in corridors, courtyard. In actuality, access is severely limited mainly because of the perceived need to control the behaviour of the children and
the overwhelming emphasis on 'therapeutic programming'.
This facility was designed with a small mudroom leading to
the outdoor recreational facilities. This room was located
at the foot of the stairs between two houses, a location
which supposedly would provide immediate and easy access to
the outdoor spaces. In addition, its amenities - a water
fountain, toilet, coat racks - would encourage the use of
the outdoor area with a minimum of inconvenience and few
staffing problems. In fact, the outdoor areas were rarely
used, except occasionally during the summer months when
children were not away on a trip. During the rest of the
year, inside 'therapeutic' programming occupied most of the
children's days. When these outdoor spaces were used, it
was for a programmed activity for a large group of children.
Use of outdoor space was viewed narrowly as 'recreation'
and 'recreation' was perceived mainly as a 'therapeutic'
tool rather than an ordinary human need. Since indoor recreational facilities were elaborate and professionally staffed
and children's behaviour was seen as potentially more con-
trollable, outdoor areas were relegated to minor importance.
The provision of a mudroom did not mean that access was
inevitable.

The addition of doors to the bedrooms and bathroom
stalls provides another example of the complex nature of
access. The director worked for three years to obtain the
money necessary for their purchase and installation. Yet
our studies show that they created only a very temporary
change in the use of bedroom and house areas and observations
indicated that the doors were open 98% of the time. Of the
2% of times the doors were closed, the rooms were usually
unoccupied. Interviews indicated that staff as well as
children viewed the doors primarily as a means of keeping
children out of unsupervised areas and safeguarding possessions even though they could not be locked. Clearly,
their physical presence and the possibilities for greater

control over use of bedrooms by the children was counteracted over time by policy decisions and practices which did not allow their use in the way intended.

Doors are viewed in a peculiar way within the context of a 'therapeutic' environment of this type. The bedroom doors are only one example. The staff's behavioural response to the installation of doors on bathroom stalls was to then keep the outer door to the bathroom open. There were doors leading to the central court from four different corridor sectors of the facility. These were always locked and the court was never used. When we renovated the seclusion rooms into dens, the staff refused to allow the door to remain solid wood and wanted a large glass panel to enable surveillance. We compromised on a very narrow glass panel which calmed fears but made surveillance difficult. Based on the definition of these children solely in terms of pathology and the expectations about their behaviour, doors may be the least therapeutic type of access mechanism. While a designer mainly views the door as a positive force, an opening leading to somewhere or a means of achieving privacy, the staff also views the same door as leading somewhere or providing privacy but in a negative context, and focuses on its need to be locked. Thus, doors usually become control mechanisms – ways of keeping children out of spaces or in the hospital. One also has to question the impact on the children of moving through a daily living environment in which virtually every door they pass by or go through is locked.

Yet, this was not always true and can be linked to the initial period of occupancy when there were so few children and staff inhabiting the 80,885 square foot building. During the first month of occupancy, the facility was used in an unstructured and spontaneous manner. Doors were unlocked and the four full care children could request and be allowed to use almost any space, any time. However, by the sixth month of occupancy with only 28 children (13 full care and 15 day care), all doors were locked, children had a programme to follow and access was highly limited. Clearly, the initial occupancy period created problems for the small staff in controlling the few children in a large space that had many doors leading to many places. Children wandered and could not be located. The response, the locking of doors, escalated over time, and did not change even when the factors creating the problem (few children, small staff) were eliminated. It is clear that the physical structure (large size, many doors, internal corridors) played a role in the continued use of this policy. However, in a setting of this type, control is always an issue - whether verbalized or not - and one incident can immediately bring it to the forefront of almost all policy decisions.

Control leads to the perception that behaviour has to be controlled, is another theme which demonstrates how changes in both physical design and policy can create institutional environments. Behaviours that one would expect to find among all children are re-interpreted because these children are seen as 'emotionally disturbed'. Running, an occasional argument, become instances of 'acting-out', and earmarked as behaviours that have to be controlled. Very often, space is used as a mechanism for control. In this hospital, one example of this theme was sending children to the house areas, called putting them 'on restriction'. If they seemed like possible runaways, they were forced to wear pajamas all day, called 'control precaution'. But the most obvious example was the rapid proliferation of seclusion rooms. Initially, there were none. In response to one or two problem incidents, one room in each house was converted into a seclusion room. Then, one room in each of the community areas was earmarked as seclusion rooms. Finally, a one-bed room in each apartment unit was made into a seclusion room. The amount of aggressive behaviour observed did not change at all during our six years of study, but the number of seclusion rooms increased tenfold. Given the present average census, there is now one seclusion room for every six children (counting day and full care).

The most overwhelming theme that emerges from the work is the regression back to the original assumptions that were basic to the State Program. Despite efforts by the architect and the director to incorporate into the design and programme qualities that would be more normalizing over time, in fact, the hospital has come to be a less and less normalized setting. In light of the labelling of these children as emotionally disabled and in need of total care, the presence of this physical structure and the concomitant social organization required to operate it inhibits the development of more human qualities and creates the institutional atmosphere.

CONCLUSIONS

While our own belief is that most children do not require residential therapy, there may always be a small group who require a supportive environment outside their home. In our research it is clear that the physical elements of such a setting can contribute to the institutional quality in a variety of functional ways (its location, size, aesthetic, internal arrangement of spaces). The physical form is a result of a way of viewing the needs of the children and the therapeutic context but it also contributes to the continuation of this view. The concrete structure must also give a message to the community, the children and the staff about the nature of people with emotional problems and the ways to deal with them. It is easy to recommend that such settings be human in scale, ordinary in its functions and aesthetics, devoid of symbols of medical treatment. More human physical settings can support the view that their inhabitants are ordinary persons. However, the physical form is not enough and our studies clearly demonstrate that it is easy to gradually slip into an institutional mode of life. Our research underlines the point that for a setting to be therapeutic, rather than institutional, it should allow its inhabitants to satisfy a variety of human needs and not constantly remind them that they are viewed as totally inadequate. Especially for children, there are a whole host of daily living experiences, e.g. putting a coin in a fare box on a bus, mailing a letter, sitting quietly and reading, which are learned only through doing them or seeing them done. We take these behaviours so for granted that it is hard to project how inadequate we would feel if we could not do them. Yet, a fairly large proportion of children are deprived of these ordinary experiences because of the nature of the physical and social settings we provide for them. What seems essential, in the future, is a broader conception of the experiences these children need and a more normalized view of the settings that should be provided for them.

REFERENCES

BETTELHEIM, B. (1974) A home for the heart, Alfred A. Knopf, New York.

GOFFMAN, E. (1959) Asylums, Aldine Press, Chicago.

HOLAHAN, C. J. and SEAGERT, S. (1973) "Psychological impact of planned environmental change: remodelling a psychiatric ward in an urban hospital", J. Abnormal Psychology, 82, pp.35-56.

HUTT, C. and VAIZEY, M. J. (1966) "Differential effects of group density on social behavior", Nature, 209, pp.1371-1372.

ITTELSON, W. H., PROSHANSKY, H. M. and RIVLIN, L. G. (1970) "Bedroom size and social interaction", Environment and Behaviour, 2, pp.255-270.

KUGEL, R. B. and WOLFENSBERGER, W. (1972) Changing patterns in residential services for the mentally retarded, US Department of Health, Education and Welfare, Social and Rehabilitation Service, Washington, DC.

RIVLIN, L. G. and WOLFE, M. (1972) "The early history of a psychiatric hospital for children: expectations and reality", Environment and Behaviour, 4, pp.33-72.

RIVLIN, L. G. (1976) "Some issues concerning institutional places", paper presented at 3rd International Architectural Psychology Conference, Univ. Louis Pasteur, Strasbourg, France, June.

TRIESCHMAN, A. E., WHITTAKER, J. K. and BRENDTRO, L. K. (1969) The other 23 hours, Aldine Pub. Co., Chicago.

WOLFE, M. (1975) "Behavioural effects of group size, room size and density in a children's psychiatric hospital", Environment and Behaviour, 7, pp.199-224.

WOLFE, M. (1977) "Environmental stimulation and design: For the 'different who are not so different'", presented at Symposium on Environmental Design for the Developmentally Disabled, Ohio State Department of Mental Health and Mental Retardation, Columbus, Ohio, April 1975. Also published in Bednar, M. J. (ed.) Barriers in the built environment, Dowden, Hutchinson, and Ross, Stroudsberg.

WOLFE, M. and GOLAN, M. B. (1976) "Privacy and Institution-alization", presented at Environmental Design Research Association Meetings, Vancouver, BC, May 1976. City University of New York Graduate School, Center for Human Environment, New York.

WOLFE, M. and RIVLIN, L. G. (1972) "Evolution of space utilization patterns in a children's psychiatric hospital", in W. Mitchell (ed.) Environmental design: research and practice, Proceedings of the EDRA III Conference, University of California at Los Angeles.

WOLFE, M., RIVLIN, L. G. and BEYDA, M. (1973) "Age-related differences in use of space", in W. Preiser (ed.) Environmental Design Research, Dowden, Hutchinson, and Ross, Stroudsberg.

Physical Environments for Autistic Children – Four Case Studies

JOHN RICHER

INTRODUCTION

This paper concerns some physical and organisational environments for the treatment of autistic children (see Rutter and Schopler, 1977, Kolvin, 1971, and Richer, 1976, for full discussions of the meaning of 'autism')[1]. The behaviour of these children is often grossly abnormal and disturbed so the question immediately arises whether the everyday physical environments and social organisations which surround most normal children are the most appropriate for the education and treatment of autistic children. Future research may reveal that manipulation of physical and social organisational environments should play only a small part in the treatment of autistic children. At the present time, however, they seem to have significant effects on behaviour which makes their investigation worthwhile.

Firstly, a note on definitions. By physical environment is meant simply, the sum total of objects that surround a child. Social organisation or social organisational environment refers to the formal structural organisation, the network of roles, in which therapy takes place, e.g. hospital, a school, a family. The above terms refer to the structures within which autistic children are treated and which are created for that treatment. Neither refers directly to the therapy itself. But particular structures, both physical and organisational, have specific implications for the type of therapy a child will receive. The knowledge of these implications must be used when planning environments.

The four environments to be described, summarised in Table 1, are not compared directly, as the necessary comparative data is not available. Each is a case study in its own right. Consideration is given to how well the physical

Table 1: Summary of four therapeutic environments

ENVIRONMENTS		I	II	III	IV
BACKGROUND	Children at outset	6 severely dis-turbed autistic children. 4 non-autistic children. Ages 4–11 years.	5 psychotic, non-speaking severely disturbed children. Ages 2½–4½ years.	3 psychotic boys. Ages 5–9 years.	1 autistic boy. Age 18 months.
	Area	Rural.	Urban.	Rural.	(Home-based).
	Previous environments	Barren hospital ward.	Home and other autistic units.	School or home	Home.
SOCIAL ORGANIZATION	Structure	Hospital.	Family/preschool.	School.	Family.
	Staff training	Nursing/other.	Teaching/nursery nurse/other.	Teaching/other.	Midwife, nursing, mal. ad. teaching. teaching.
	Staff:child ratio	Between 1:1 and 1:10	1:1	1:1	Mother (plus therapist):child.

TABLE 1 (continued)

ENVIRONMENTS	I	II	III	IV
SOCIAL ORGANIZATION — Therapy programmes (see text for further details) — AIMS	To increase social interactions and decrease social avoidance.	To decrease avoidance, teach skills e.g. language.	To decrease avoidance and teach social and academic skills.	To increase attachment between mother and child.
METHODS	Relaxed non-intrusive behaviour. Interact in way child suggests.	Complex: initially fostering attachment, in relaxed accepting atmosphere then gradual teaching of skills (but see text).	Have tutors with child in classroom and elsewhere. Standard teaching procedures plus special activities e.g. music therapy.	Reduce verbal/visual intrusiveness and increase body contact/baby games. Slow down pace of interaction.
PHYSICAL ENVIRONMENT	Robust safe playroom. Soft area, long soft seats, activity house, fixed tables and benches, lockable cupboards.	Many rooms with different functions e.g. skills training, bath, eating, cooking, painting, creative play; staff discussion and relaxation.	In primary school. (Elliott cabin with craft facilities, quiet area, one way screen, office, tables).	Home. Reduced use of mother aids (increased body contact).

TABLE 1 (continued)

ENVIRONMENTS		I	II	III	IV
EVALUATION	AFTER	5 years.	2 years.	3 years.	1 year.
	Behaviour change	More social interactions, fewer stereotypies, but no dramatic improvements.	2 children speaking and going to primary school. Others sociable and showing great improvement.	None showing severe autistic behaviour. All integrated into school, speaking, reading, 1 child to secondary school part-time.	Great increase in attachment and decrease in avoidance. Some words.

environment and the social organisation of the therapeutic
unit complement each other and how appropriate the total
system is to the treatment of autistic children. In each
case one important consideration is the degree to which the
system differs from the everyday environments of normal
children and whether these deviations from the everyday,
which are intended to promote therapy, in fact do so.

ENVIRONMENT I - A HOSPITAL WARD PLAYROOM

This playroom, which was designed by S. Nicoll and
myself, has been described elsewhere (Richer and Nicoll,
1971) so I shall only outline the project. The playroom
was built in the ward day area of a hospital for autistic
and emotionally disturbed children. The ward contained 10
children aged between 4 and 11 years. Six were autistic,
conforming to Kanner's syndrome (Kanner, 1943), the others
were severely disturbed but not autistic. The ward was
staffed by nurses or nursing assistants. The staff/child
ratio varied between 1:1 and 1:10, depending upon the time
of day. All the children were at school or other training
sessions from 9.30 to 11.45 and from 1.30 to 3.30. For the
rest of the time they were in the care of the nurses, although they were not always in the ward. The ward was
therefore their 'home' room, and little or no formal instruction was intended to take place there.

The ward before conversion

Before conversion, the ward was furnished with tables,
chairs and a few cupboards. The children were continually
being stopped from doing things for fear they would hurt
themselves or destroy the furniture. There were few toys
around, since those put out, being inadequate, were soon
broken. It was even difficult for a child to sit on someone's lap, since most of the chairs were narrow and had hard
arms. In the dining room, the chairs and tables were easily
moved around, which made a lot of noise; a child sitting at
a table might have it pushed into his stomach by the child
opposite him; the children often jumped up and ran round.

The children were frustrated and highly avoiding. They
were, in effect, over-crowded, and people were mainly
sources of frustration. This did not reduce the autistic
children's avoidance, neither was it an easy or rewarding
environment for staff to work in, which in turn affected the
quality of care they gave the children. The new playroom
attempted to remedy these faults and construct a positive
therapeutic environment.

The new playroom

The playroom is illustrated in Figure 1. Some of the means by which we tried to remedy the faults of the old playroom and decrease autistic children's tendency to avoid social interactions were as follows:

1. All structures were robust, safe and easily cleaned, staff did not continually have to stop the children from doing things for fear they might hurt themselves or damage furniture in the room. All cupboards were lockable to prevent breakage of televisions, radios, etc.

2. The area was divided into connected parts by the existing walls, the activity house and the blackboard. This reduced the avoidance-provoking effects of others, in effect it reduced over-crowding.

3. Autistic children are agile, dextrous and rarely hurt themselves by accident. Moreover, they seem to enjoy activities like climbing, sliding, etc. The activity house met these requirements. It was also an enclosed area which might put a child in close proximity to another, but at a time when each was enjoying himself; so that, we hoped, avoidance behaviour would be less likely and social interaction more likely.

4. The social contact and interaction most autistic children usually seek is of two sorts: they seek close tactile contact, sitting on people's laps, clinging closely and avoiding eye contact, or alternatively, they may seek rough-and-tumble play, wanting to be swung around, lifted up, tickled, etc. The long low soft seats and soft pad allowed cuddling to take place easily and comfortably and the pad could be used for rough and tumble play.

5. The noise and movement at meal-times had often escalated into 'epidemics of disturbance'. To reduce the frequency of these, the children sat on a continuous bench surrounding each table, and both tables and benches were fixed to the floor. This inhibited swivelling, jumping up and running around.

Instructions to staff

The intention behind the playroom was explained to staff and they were told that they need not stop children doing things (including stereotypies) because the room was safe, robust and easy to clean. Any cupboards they wanted

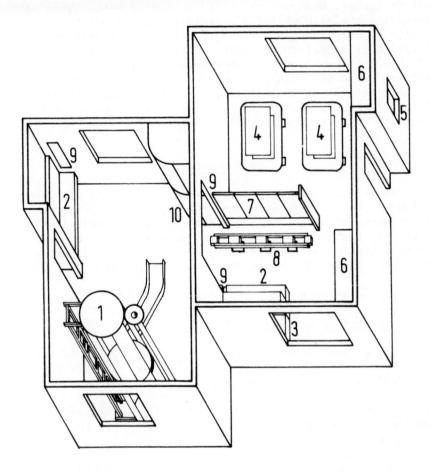

Figure 1: Axonometric of Environment I

1. Activity house
2. Soft seats
3. Soft pad
4. Fixed tables and continuous benches
5. Serving hatch from kitchen
6. Lockable cupboards containing TV, radio, record player, toys, etc.
7. 'Stimulus' wall and blackboard
8. Walkway
9. Mirrors (some facing each other)
10. Retreat box, hideaway

to lock could be locked. They were asked to make very few
approaches to the children, but to wait until the child
approached. At that point they should interact, doing,
within limits, whatever the child seemed to want. Thus we
hoped the autistic children's avoidance would not be stimulated by over-intense adult approaches, and that the
duration of social interactions would be enhanced, because
(1) the child would be approach-motivated (he had, after
all, made the approach), (2) staff would not be too reactive
to him, and (3) he would be doing something he could do.
We hoped the experience of rewarding social encounters would
increase the frequency of social interactions.

Evaluation

Behaviours were time-sampled: (1) in the old playroom
a few months before conversion, and (2) in the new playroom
a few weeks after conversion. Recordings were made in the
free play sessions after lunch and before tea, 4 records
being taken for each child at each time, with the constraint
that the child was not observed twice during any one period.

The behaviours time-sampled were as follows:

1.   Stereotyped activities and postures.

2.   Social approaches to another child or adult. Behaviour,
such as looking at another person, could not be reliably
assessed, so it was not scored.

3.   Interaction with another person. In this category,
one person must not be merely passive, each must react to
the other.

4.   Object manipulation of the physical environment, such
as toys, fixtures, structures, etc.

Results

Data for the 6 autistic children were separated from
that of the 4 non-autistic children. The results are shown
in Figure 2 and were as follows:

1.   Stereotyped behaviours were less frequent in the new
playroom.

2.   Interactions were more frequent in the new playroom.

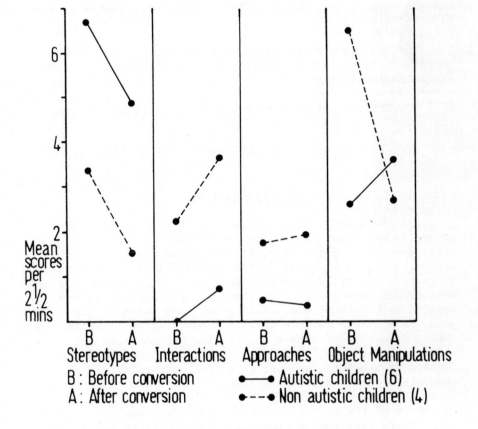

Figure 2: Evaluation of Environment I

Mean scores per 2½ minutes of behaviours time sampled
before and after conversion

3.   Approaches and object manipulation showed no significant change.   However, these were the less reliable measures.

These results were interesting in view of the instructions given to staff, namely, not to approach the children and not to stop stereotypies. The results were in the direction we predicted.

The time sampling measures also differentiated between the six children in the autistic group and the other children, in the following ways:

1.   Stereotyped behaviours were more frequent in the autistic group.

2.   Interactions were less frequent in the autistic group.

Other observations

The children's general behaviour in the room was observed.   Some 'territoriality' developed.   For instance, one girl spent most of her time, for the first three or four months, lying on the seat in the alcove.   When anybody approached she tried to push them away.   She occasionally made forays into the rest of the room, but when upset retreated to this seat and, rolling back and forth on her side, soon quietened down if left alone.   After 6 months she no longer spent such a lot of time on that seat but mixed more with other children, gave people much more eye contact than before, and delighted her parents by greeting them with eye contact and smiling.

Most of the structures were used in the ways we expected.   There were some exceptions.   For the first six months the retreat box was hardly used.   One girl went in fleetingly to leave things there, but no one stayed for any length of time.   Some swung on the door.   Then one 6 year old autist took a small dog on rockers in there and stayed in there for long periods with the door closed.   If the door was opened by another child he could be seen sitting on the dog and perhaps rocking.

The PVC covers did not turn out to be bite-proof, and one was ripped.   However, assaults on covers ceased after one week, for about a year, although eventually the covers had to be renewed (twice).

The dining area has been successful in cutting down such behaviours as jumping up and running away, throwing water and food around, and tantrums. Mealtimes passed off more smoothly and quietly. This was often helped by playing a 'soothing' record quietly during meals.

The most successful area was the soft pad. This attracted a lot of children, especially in the evenings when the lights are dimmed or out, and only a green spotlight played on the pad from above, and perhaps the television was on. They curled up amongst fur coats, cushions, adults and each other. They were quiet, close to each other, and yet seemed relaxed. It is a fair hypothesis that they were learning to be close to other people and relaxed at the same time. This has obvious parallels with relaxation/desensitisation therapy (cf. Graziano and Kean, 1968).

The ward sister noted great changes in the behaviour of some of the children after 6 months. Some of the six autists tolerated being close to other people for long periods without becoming unduly tense, they sometimes engaged in eye contact for as long as ten seconds. They played simple tickling and stroking games and solicited these, some even made approaches to other children, with eye contact (and without the aim of, for instance, snatching something away) and perhaps played touching or chasing games or just touched the other child in an exploratory way. All this was virtually unknown before the regime.

Postscript

The playroom was intended as the physical precondition for successful therapy given hospital organisation and values. It was quite successful in increasing social interactions and reducing stereotypies, but none of the autistic children could be described as recovered, and it is instructive to enquire why. One answer lies in the children themselves: none spoke or had high IQs before the age of 5, which makes their prognosis poor (Kanner, 1971, Rutter, 1974). However, an equally interesting reason may be sought in the nature of the hospital's formal organisational structure. This is a hierarchy in which the people who work with the children ('contact' people) are not the ones who make the major decisions. In addition, there is a proliferation of professionals working with a child and each does not have enough time to communicate adequately with all the others. These problems are discussed in the next section, before we go on to discuss the other three environments.

Autistic children and the family

To the biologist versed in evolutionary theory, the fact that most children are reared in families suggests that both children and adults are well adapted to such a social organisation. This is hardly a novel thought but one which is frequently forgotten when that organisation breaks down. Like any biological system, each family has its tolerance limits to stress and these limits are often exceeded when the family contains an autistic child, so that child is taken out of the family and put in an institution like unit I's hospital. Like the family, the institution feeds and protects the child, but other aspects of family-like organisation are often absent, partly because the child disrupts that very organisation.

What are these other aspects? One, long recognised, is that the child and the few adults that care for him become attached to each other (Bowlby, 1971) and, in our culture, the child seems especially attached to its mother in the early years. Autistic children, on the other hand, do not show the same attachment behaviour towards their parents as other children. They give the impression of being unattached, which makes mothering difficult.

Another aspect, less often stated and perhaps taken for granted, is that parents are free to react intuitively and spontaneously to their children. From an intimate and subtle knowledge of their child, gained largely from first hand experience, they react to their children, in the context of their goals and ideals, according to the subtleties and complexities of the immediate situation. They rarely react on the basis of verbal instructions or explicit theory. Relationships between parents and children are progressively and continually negotiated in social interactions. Autistic children, however, tend to avoid social interactions. People feel that autistic children do not form emotional relationships, that they do not communicate. We are often confused as our 'normal' behaviour just does not seem to 'work'. The child does not develop at an acceptable rate and remains socially avoiding (i.e. autistic).

From this, and from autistic children's other problems such as gross temper tantrums and destructiveness it is little wonder that an autistic child puts a severe strain on his family and that many are sent to hospital. Yet such places, as King, Raynes and Tizard (1971) have valuably explained, are organised in an 'institution-oriented' way; they tend to put organisational needs before those of the child. There are set routines and clear hierarchies. Junior staff, who are most in contact with the children, have little freedom to react spontaneously. Staff are moved from ward to ward frequently. Staff turnover is high so there is little chance for staff to gain a really comprehensive and intuitive knowledge of the children, and, even if they did, there is little opportunity to use it, since instructions are handed down the hierarchy, often emanating from people who know less about the child than the junior person with first hand experience. Instructions are often inadequate as it is one thing to prescribe a certain drug dosage, but quite another to specify the subtleties of social behaviour. Social interactions are unfolding negotiations and are very difficult to predict, let alone prescribe. On top of this, even when someone sincerely believes himself to be acting according to instructions he may be observed interacting in a very different way. Elusive qualities like his personality and the exact nature of the unfolding situation seem at least as important as stated instructions.

This institution orientation also protects staff from becoming attached to the children, and vice versa. The staff in an institution-oriented unit can cope with the attachment difficulties and confusions generated by autistic children because their work is often more directed towards running the organisation, than developing the child. Even in advanced hospitals a child is seen by so many different professionals that a comprehensive understanding of the child and goals of treatment is not fully developed since the professionals seldom have time to communicate with each other or see each other at work. Social interactions, the negotiation of relationships, the transmission of culture, and the ideals and goals of parents, are all so complex and subtle, that the proper development of a child, especially an autistic child, can perhaps be best achieved when the adults have first hand knowledge of the children and are able to interact intuitively and spontaneously. This happens in the family. We are left with a paradox; autistic children's own families, or family like units, often cannot cope with them, yet the institutions which can, do so at the cost of aspects of family social organisation which are probably vital to a child's development. It seems we need a social organisation which preserves some vital attributes of the family but also has qualities which allow adults to cope with the stress and confusion generated by autistic children and at the same time treat and educate them.

ENVIRONMENT II: A UNIT FOR PRESCHOOL AUTISTIC CHILDREN

There have been many attempts to solve this problem in
the past. One recent attempt is a unit in North London.
It now has 7 children diagnosed autistic, aged between 2½
and 4½ years, on referral. The maximum number of children
the unit will accept is 9. The children arrive at 9.30 and
leave at 3.30. There is a 1:1 staff/child ratio; each
member of staff commits him or herself to stay for at least
2 years.

Social organisation

Having carefully selected her staff the Director allows
them considerable autonomy. As in a family, staff have
freedom to react spontaneously to the child in each new
situation. This is possible because the adults develop a
comprehensive and subtle intuitive knowledge of each child
from first hand experience. They are also aware of what
everybody else is doing with a child from discussion, and,
again, from first hand experience. Consistent staff attitudes towards children, parents, and each other are developed
in continual informal discussions and in lengthy group meetings once a week. In this way, some of the preconditions
for the consistent and sensitive treatment which a child
might expect in a family are developed. Such consistency
is especially necessary with autistic children since their
reaction to even the slightest confusion is often extreme
social avoidance and stereotyped behaviour.

A concomitant of this freedom is great flexibility,
allowing an adult to interact with a child for five minutes
or five hours, depending on the circumstances. The staff
can capitalise on a child's interest, just as a mother might
with her normal infant, catching the child's interest on
the flood and developing it. Again, this is especially
necessary with autistic children who are much more reluctant
than normal children to accept tasks presented to them.

The flexibility allows staff to carry through a task
to completion. Autistic children tend to give up directed
activities at the slightest difficulty, and immediately try
to avoid further social contact. However, provided the
task is skillfully chosen to be within the child's competence, the adult can persist uninterrupted until the task
is eventually done. At this unit the children have now
gained confidence that things started will be completed
successfully. The relationship, negotiated between child
and adult in successful interactions, becomes more positive

and trusting, which further promotes new learning. Throughout, the child has to act himself, and the adult waits for
him to do so; if a child runs away from an activity the
adult waits for him to come back, but makes it clear that
the coming back is what is expected. At some units, a child
wishing to stop the interaction, might become destructive
and would then be sent out of the room. But in this unit,
this is seen as collusion in, and reinforcement of, the
child's destructiveness and social avoidance, and the child
would not be sent out, but expected to complete the task.

Autistic children are very easily distracted from their
work. Teachers in charge of more than one child frequently
have their attention drawn from the child they are working
with by the disruption of another child. The 1:1 staff-child
ratio helps prevent this.

Physical environment

Many units for autistic children work in just one room.
This unit has 6 main therapy rooms (Figure 3) which, like
the 1:1 staff-child ratio, helps reduce distractions. An
interaction between an adult and a child is, of course,
respected by other adults who do not intrude; the children
too, after a few months, come to respect such interactions,
to such an extent that the internal doors in the unit were
removed.

Different areas of a child's development are reflected
in different rooms as follows.

1. Skills room — with Montessori and other equipment for quiet maths and language
   work.

2. Activity room — with a Wendy house, toys and
   painting materials for creative
   play.

3. Music room — with piano, bells, xylophones,
   drums, etc. This unit employs a
   music teacher.

4. Kitchen — staff and children lunch together.

5. Lounge — for staff discussion and a quiet
   time after lunch with staff and
   children together.

78

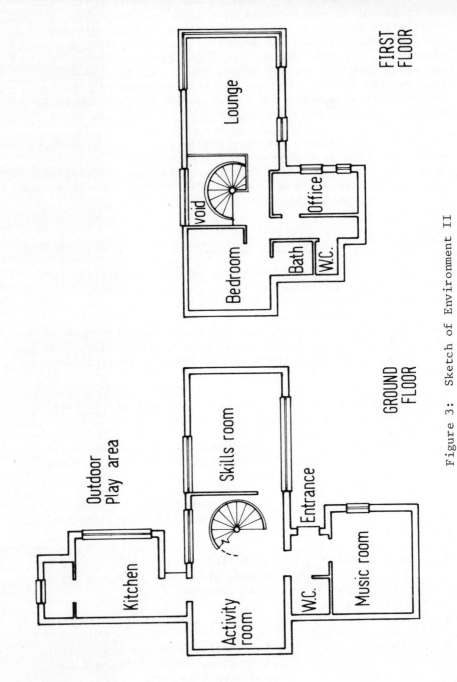

Figure 3: Sketch of Environment II

6.   Bedroom/bathroom   baths can last as long as 2 hours
                            and provide a valuable relaxing
                            medium for playful and educative
                            social interaction.

Observing where a child goes gives valuable clues about
the kind of activity he wants, and interestingly, during
their first few months at the unit, children went mostly to
the skills room, spending up to four hours a day there,
suggesting they preferred that more structured setting.

Evaluation

Five children attended the school in its first two
years. From being severely autistic and not speaking, two
children now attend normal primary school and speak. All
five children now show very little of the predominant social
avoidance and stereotyped behaviour characteristic of autistic children. All have gained greatly in general competence.

ENVIRONMENT III: AN AUTISTIC UNIT IN A PRIMARY SCHOOL

This unit for autistic children is set in a rural primary school. The essential environmental feature of this
unit is simply that it is in a school. This brings two huge
benefits:

1.   The autistic children have normal peers to imitate.

2.   The autistic children have to learn to adapt to the
social organisation and social behaviour of normal children.
This contrasts with units exclusively for disturbed children,
where each child has only the disturbed behaviour of the
others to imitate and adapt to. It is little wonder that
such children are slow in acquiring 'normal' social behaviour
patterns.

The essential organisational feature of this unit
(apart from being in a school) is that each child has a
'home tutor' with him in the school classroom. This helps
protect the rest of the class from any disruption that the
autistic child might cause, as well as providing him with
individual attention.

This scheme in fact started by accident when the school
headmaster had reluctantly to exclude a 6 year old boy from
school, because he was so disruptive in class. Thus, he

was then receiving no education, so a home tutor was appointed. After working with this boy a short while, the home tutor asked if she could bring him back into school if she guaranteed he would not disrupt the class. After that, two more autistic boys were brought into the scheme and more home tutors were employed.

After this scheme had been operating for about four years, it was decided that the autistic children would benefit from having their own room in which activities like music therapy and pottery, as well as individual teaching, could take place. In addition, the room was to be a 'home' room. However, the children still went to classes with other children and played in the playground. An Elliot cabin was purchased and the author was asked to design the interior in consultation with the teachers and consultant psychiatrist. The result is shown in Figure 4. It must be emphasised, however, that there is nothing exceptional about this room itself. The essential environmental feature is that the unit is <u>in a primary school</u>.

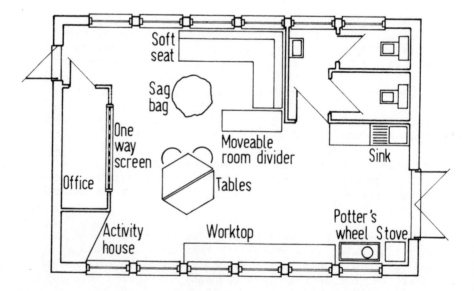

Figure 4: Sketch plan of interior of Elliot cabin. (There are 2 movable room dividers and 4 trapezium shaped tables in the hut. One room divider has a blackboard, the other a pinboard, on the back.) Remember the most important feature of the physical environment is that the unit is in a primary school.

Table 2: Psychological test results of first three boys in Environment III

	AGE IN YEARS AND MONTHS	TEST RESULTS
Boy 1	5+	Entered project.
	6.5	Reynell[1] comprehension age 4.0 yrs expressive language age 4.5 yrs
	7.2	Reynell comprehension age 4.3 yrs expressive language age 6.0 yrs
	11.1	WISC IQ[2] F:78 V:69 P:93 Neale[3] Accuracy level 10.1 yrs Comprehension level 8.8 yrs
Boy 2	4.5	Vineland[5] Social age 2.6 yrs
	5.3	Said to be untestable on IQ tests but thought to be functioning at approximately a 2½ year level.
	6.4	Again could not be properly tested but thought to be functioning at a 3 year level. Speech echolalic. Very poor concentration. Entered project.
	11.8	WISC IQ F:72 V:56 P:57 Neale Accuracy level 7.10 yrs Comprehension level 6.9 yrs
Boy 3[6]	8.4	Stanford Binet IQ: 56
	9.3	Entered project. Stanford Binet IQ: 46
	10.9	WISC IQ F:48 V:60 P:46
	13.11	WISC IQ F:64 V:74 P:61 Neale Accuracy level 10.5 yrs Comprehension level 8.10 yrs

Table 2 (cont.)

1.   Reynell Developmental language scales

2.   Wechsler Intelligence Scale for Children

        F = Full Scale IQ
        V = Verbal IQ
        P = Performance IQ

3.   Neale Analysis of Reading Ability

4.   Stanford Binet Intelligence Test

5.   Vineland Social Maturity Scale

6.   The progress of boy 3 must be set against the doubt
       that the original diagnosis of autism was correct.
       However, he was extremely disturbed and retarded.

Evaluation

The progress of the first three boys to take part in
this project is shown in Table 2. The behaviour of all
three boys is greatly improved; they are vastly more sociable
and socially acceptable than before. They now concentrate
well on school work. None would now be described as autistic.
The oldest now attends secondary school part-time and the
progress of all is sufficient to justify an optimistic
prognosis.

ENVIRONMENT IV: A HOME BASED TREATMENT PROGRAMME

The concept of home-based treatment for autistic children illustrates further the point made earlier concerning
the degree of deviation from everyday (normal) environments
necessary for treatment.

Home-based programmes have two essential features:

1.   Environmental feature; treatment takes place at home.

2.   Organizational feature; the parents, usually the mother,
       are the agents for the treatment.

Since the treatment setting is the everyday environment
of the family, the problems encountered by conventional
treatments of generalization to that everyday physical and

social environment do not exist.

Howlin et al (1973) conducted an interesting language teaching programme based on a behaviour modification approach with good results. The author is currently evaluating a home-based programme for autistic children under 2 years old, where the initial aim is to increase the attachment between mother and child. The therapist visits the home once a week and offers suggestions to the mother, based on her observations of what the mother is doing to promote attachment. From the point of view of this paper some interesting environmental points have emerged. Designers might note that the therapist has found herself recommending that the mother reduces her use of certain aids, such as a changing-board or high chair, because they inhibit attachment between mother and child. For instance, one mother used to change her child on a changing board, set on top of a cot. This is efficient and acceptable for normal children. However, since the board was so high it was difficult for mother and child ever to establish eye contact should the child want it. This is a serious handicap for a child so tenuously attached. In fact, the mother was asked to change the child on her lap, and to feed him on her lap, to soap him prior to bathing on her lap, and to carry him around on her hip. Here then the use of special environmental or physical aids is minimized in order to increase attachment between the young autistic child and his mother. This particular boy is now 2 years old and has so far made very good progress; he is less avoiding, more sociable and is saying a few words.

Interestingly, by maximizing close physical contact between the child and mother, the mother's role in this respect approaches that seen in modern hunter-gatherer societies (Blurton Jones, 1976). Perhaps our cultural evolution has come full circle in this respect, such that a therapeutic environment for a young autistic child is similar to an infant's normal environment in some 'primitive' cultures. This has important implications for more institutional settings, in that the over-provision of modern environmental aids may prevent the necessary interpersonal contact for the child's progress.

CONCLUSIONS

These four case studies illustrate some possible physical and social organizational environments for autistic children. All have yet to be adequately evaluated, but it may be safely said that the latter three are superior to the first. In Environment IV, the autistic children were infants, in II they were pre-school age, and in III they were school age, but in all three cases the deviation from the everyday physical and social organizational environments of like aged normal children was less than in I. The task for the future is perhaps to find these minimal deviations necessary for adequate therapy. This sounds obvious but the needs of institutions and professions have sometimes led us away from this simple maxim.

Footnote

[1] The view of autistic children (Kanner, 1943; Kolvin, 1971; Rutter, 1974) implicit in this paper is, very briefly, this. Autistic children avoid social interactions much more than non autistic children (Richer, 1976). This avoidance is decreased by generally not looking much or intensely reacting to the child initially (Richer and Coss, 1976; Richer and Richards, 1975) and by avoiding difficult or uncertain activities (Churchill, 1971; Richer, 1978). Intense avoidance helps retard acquisition of language and other social skills (Richer, 1973, 1978). The initial main aims of therapy are to reduce social avoidance, promote communicating relationships, and develop social skills, including language.

REFERENCES

BLURTON JONES, J. (1976) <u>Ecological aspects of the biology of mother-infant interaction</u>, paper presented in Human Ethology Sumposium, B.P.S. Annual Conference, York.

BOWLBY, J. (1971) <u>Attachment</u>, Penguin, Harmondsworth.

CHURCHILL, D. W. (1971) "The effects of success and failure in psychotic children", <u>Arch. Gen. Psychiat.</u>, 25, pp.208-214.

GRAZIANO, A. M. and KEAN, J. E. (1968) "Programmed relaxation and reciprocal inhibition with psychotic children", <u>Behav. Res. Ther.</u>, 6, pp.433-437.

HOWLIN, P., MARCHANT, R., RUTTER, M., BERGER, M., HERSOV, L., and YULE, W. (1973) "A home-based approach to the treatment of autistic children", <u>J. Aut. Child. Schiz.</u>, 34, pp.308-336.

HUTT, C. (1969) "Exploration, arousal and autism", <u>Psychol. Forsch.</u>, 33, pp.1-8.

KANNER, L. (1943) "Autistic disturbances of affective contact", <u>Nerv. Child</u>, 2, pp.217-250.

KANNER, L. (1971) "Follow up study of 11 autistic children originally reported in 1943", <u>J. Aut. Child. Schiz.</u>, 1, pp.119-145.

KING, R., RAYNES, N., and TIZARD, J. (1971) <u>Patterns of residential care</u>, Routledge and Kegan Paul.

KOLVIN, I. (1971) "Diagnostic criteria and classification of childhood psychosis", <u>Brit. J. Psychiat.</u>, 118, pp.381-384.

RICHER, J. M. and NICOLL, S. (1971) "A playroom for autistic children and its companion therapy project", Brit. J. Ment. Subnormality, 17, pp.132-143.

RICHER, J. M. (1973) Some effects of autistic children's social behaviour on their learning and development, paper read at B.P.S. London Conference.

RICHER, J. M. and RICHARDS, B. (1975) "Reacting to autistic children - the danger of trying too hard", Brit. J. Psychiat., 127, pp.526-529.

RICHER, J. M. and COSS, R. G. (1976) "Gaze aversion in autistic and normal children", Acta. Psychiat. Scand., 53, pp.193-210.

RICHER, J. M. (1976) "The social avoidance behaviour of autistic children", Anim. Behav., 24, pp.898-906.

RICHER, J. M. (1978) "The partial non-communication of culture to autistic children", in Autism: A reappraisal of concepts and treatment, M. Rutter and E. Schopler (eds.), Plenum Press.

RUTTER, M. (1974) "The development of infantile autism", Psychol. Med., 4, pp.147-163.

The Adventure Playground as a Therapeutic Environment

PAUL WOLFF

PLAY AND THE HANDICAPPED CHILD

Many handicapped children spend a disproportionate part of their time in some type of structured environment, such as a school or institution, where play tends to be structured, organized and restricted. Such children have been shown to be particularly slow in language development and social skills (W. Dennis, et al, 1957). Michael Ellis (1973) has defined the problem concisely by stating that "Handicaps work a cruel double blow to the development of an individual. They limit the potential of the individual and they handicap the process whereby the person achieves his potential...The ill and handicapped human has greater need for recreation or play services because their limited circumstances to some extent prevent their exploring for opportunities themselves".

In order to explore the various aspects of play behaviour in relation to the physical and social parameters in which they are free to occur, I spent several months in 1974 comparing two radically different play environments and the social behaviours stimulated by each in children with a specific physical handicap - that of severely impaired vision (Wolff, 1975).

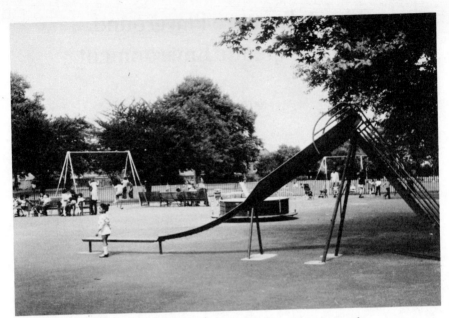

Figure 1: The Conventional Playground

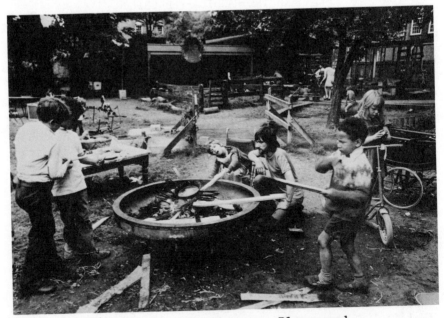

Figure 2: The Adventure Playground

It is not actually defective vision or any additional handicaps that ultimately are the dominant force restraining the child's progress and development. Rather, it is the physiological and psychological effect that this condition creates on him and on those with whom he comes into contact. It is this that determines his ultimate potential. The ability and self-assurance to effectively communicate with others is a vital factor in determining this effect. The visually defective child may experience early difficulties in the use of all three essential components of communication - speech, language, and play (Scholl in Lowenfeld, 1973).

Play is possibly the most essential means of communication (Winnicot, 1971), especially for the very young. It can help to promote personal confidence in relations with others. It can serve to minimize the poverty of environmental information to which they have access by promoting exploration and manipulation through experimentation. Auditory input alone, being devoid of experience, has only limited potential to convey information. Play can help the child to realize that he has the ability to cause a change in the environment and thereby communicate something about himself. In short, play allows each individual to obtain personally significant meaning from his environment through direct physical and social interaction. This implies, however, that the play setting must contain sufficient information, novelty and complexity to facilitate and stimulate such interaction. Thus, play takes on far greater significance for the visually handicapped child than for the sighted, particularly in relation to social development (Huffman, 1957).

THE SPECIFIC PLAY ENVIRONMENTS

This paper compares the influence of the physical and social characteristics of two distinct types of play environments - a conventional playground (CPG) and an adventure playground (APG) - on the social and non-social aspects of play of the same four to five year old and seven to ten year old visually handicapped children. Unobtrusive time sampling observations were used to record the frequency of activity changes as well as the frequencies of six mutually exclusive types of play behaviour (definitions adapted from Jones, 1972).

1. Solitary play (Figure 3): an activity engaged in alone, without interaction with another or cue from another.

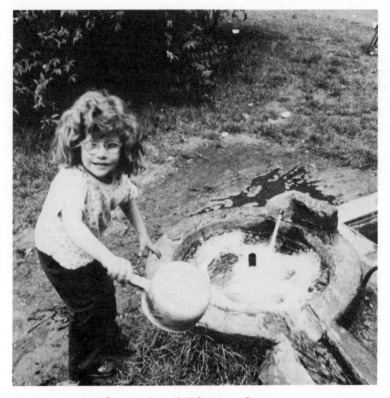

Figure 3: Solitary play

2. Parallel Play (Figure 4): engaging in a similar activ-
    ity to another without interacting with that person.
    Activity normally occurs near other person without
    verbal or physical contact, i.e. sand play, on swings
    or slides.

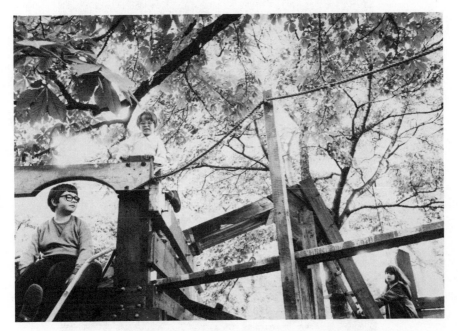

Figure 4: Parallel play

3. Positive Interaction with Peer (Figure 5): Piaget
    (Flavell, 1963) has noted that meaningful cooperative
    play does not usually occur prior to the age of seven
    or eight. Nevertheless, a play activity can readily
    be dominated by positive or negative interaction with
    either peer or adult at the age of four or five (Wright,
    1960). This is frequently, though not always, accom-
    panied by verbal behaviour, i.e. conversation (friendly),
    pushing each other on swing or car, going down slide
    interwined, climbing together while conversing, holding
    hands, helping one another, etc.

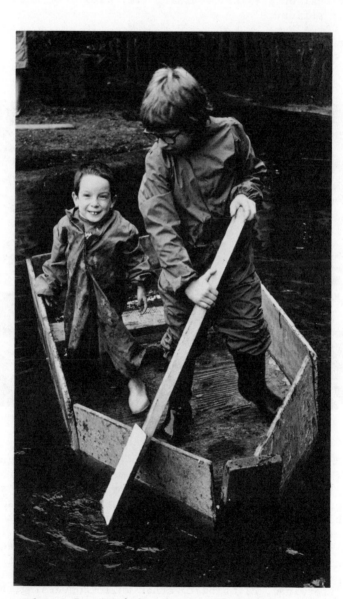

Figure 5: Positive interaction with peers

4. Negative Interaction with Peers: this category would include aggressive behaviour (i.e. fighting, arguing), non-cooperation, resisting or avoiding interaction with a peer, ignoring or refusing to comply with or accept a social approach of a peer (Wright, 1960).

5. Positive Interaction with Adults (Figure 6): cooperating with an adult, receiving or offering assistance.

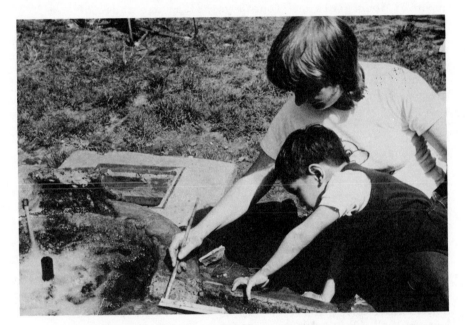

Figure 6: Positive Interaction with Adults

6. Negative Interaction with Adults: non-cooperative behaviour with an adult, aggressive behaviour (fighting, kicking, screaming), resisting help, resisting interaction.

The observed changes of activity signified a distinct change of emphasis from one activity to another. If a change in response was an integral part of a behaviour sequence, it was not classified as a change of activity. For example, a child climbing a ladder to get to the top of a slide was not recorded as a different activity from sliding down the slide, if the latter followed immediately after the former. However, if the child after climbing to the top of the slide sat there to talk with another child or merely observed the actions of others, the behaviour qualified as a change of activity. Similarly, if one child joined another in cooperative sand play, it was still the same activity. Only if the two children then embarked on a different activity, e.g. tumbling in the sand, filling each other's pockets with sand, etc., was it then noted as a change of activity.

The younger children consisted of three girls and four boys ranging in age from 4.5 to 5.7 years, while the older group of four girls and four boys had an age range of 7.6 to 10.4. All the children attended a London special school for the partially seeing on a full-time basis. They were taken to each of the two playgrounds once a week, for a period of one hundred and five minutes. Five one-minute time units were grouped together to constitute one five-minute observation period. Two such five-minute periods in random non-sequential order were recorded for each child during each visit to the playground. In this way, the behaviour of each child was recorded for two series of five one-minute observations in each of four weekly sessions - giving a total of forty one-minute observations per child at each playground. The seven to ten year olds were not taken to the conventional playground as these facilities were found to be "too boring" (comment of a student) by the class and too inactive by the teacher. Instead, this group spent their equivalent play time engaged in organized ball games (using a ball with a bell in it) on the large grass area adjacent to the conventional playground. Organized ball games are not a free choice play situation and were not considered to be valid activities for the chosen social behavioural categories. "Play is unrestricted, while games have rules" (Opie, 1969). Therefore the activities of the older group of students were only recorded when they were at the adventure playground, and can only be compared to the younger group's behaviour in the same setting.

Two types of playgrounds

A conventional playground and an adventure playground were chosen to represent two basic strongly contrasting concepts of play behaviour which contained a minimum of direct adult influence for this particular user group.

The term conventional playground as used here refers to play areas most commonly operated by local public authorities, which are often part of a community or neighbourhood park and which contain a variety of fixed play equipment.

This equipment, of durable metal construction, typically comprises mass-produced catalogue items such as slides, swings, climbing apparatus, etc. The ground surface normally consists of a non-resilient material such as asphalt paving. Low maintenance is a prime design criterion of these facilities, since they do not usually provide any type of adult play leadership. These playgrounds which abound in most urban western societies have remarkably similar physical characteristics, although a variety of terms is used to describe them, e.g. traditional, equipped, or conventional playground, paved play area, asphalt jungle, etc.

In contrast, adventure playgrounds are defined by reference to the activities they provide for rather than by their physical appearance. In London, which presently contains approximately 86 such playgrounds, the Adventure Playground Association uses the operational definition of "a place where children of all ages, under friendly supervision, are free to do many things they can no longer easily do in our crowded urban society - things like building dens, tree houses, huts; lighting fires and cooking; climbing, digging, camping, gardening, painting, dressing-up, reading - or doing nothing" (London Adventure Playground Association, 1972).

The physical facilities can vary considerably depending upon economic factors as well as local interest and involvement. Basic essentials typically consist of a play hut containing storage space, indoor play space, toilets, phone and play-leaders office; building materials such as wood, nails, rope, tires, bricks, etc.; tools (hammers, saws, chisels, etc.); materials for dressing up, painting, clay modelling, etc.; and sturdy fencing enclosing the entire area.

The historical development and public acceptance of the conventional and adventure playground differ radically (Bengtsson, 1972; Lady Allen, 1955; Benjamin, 1966); but there are also fundamental differences in the objectives of both types of playground. These differences come most sharply into focus if we consider the information content of the environment in relation to the types of play behaviour that each environment stimulates. The information content of the conventional playground implies a static, permanent adult structured facility, with only the presence of the users themselves providing for change, variety, novelty or complexity. It provides for extrinsically motivated physical play activities, involving coordinated motor skills and large muscle development.

Since both the spirit and the activities of an adventure playground are often heavily influenced by its immediate neighbourhood, a blanket description becomes more difficult. Most adventure playgrounds, however, provide for play as intrinsically motivated arousal-seeking behaviour. They attempt to create a dynamic, constantly changing play setting, which promotes active participation through the use of novel, varied and complex stimuli.

The children remained the same (or did they?), only the play settings to which they were exposed changed. What, therefore, were the specific physical and social character-istics of each playground?

The conventional playground (Figure 1)

The conventional playground occupied .43 acre within a pleasant 5.5 acres typical London urban park. The park was surrounded on three sides by late 19th century terraced and semi-detached housing. The major portion of the fourth side was taken up by the elementary school, an austere looking four-storey brick edifice built around the turn of the century. The playground was in the far-western corner of this park, surrounded by a four-foot high iron picket fence. Dispersed upon its tarmacadam surface, under two large oak trees, were located seven pieces of galvanized steel play equipment, several wooden benches and a small covered seating area between two small structures containing toilet facilities. The fixed equipment consisted of a ten-foot diameter swingabout (a ten-foot high central steel column), three straight slides of varying heights, a ten-foot diameter roundabout and two sets of four swings each.

The adventure playground (Figure 2)

In area, the adventure playground was remarkably similar to the conventional playground, covering roughly .45 acre, within the three acres comprising the "second largest privately-owned garden in London" (Handicapped Adventure Playground Association, 1973). The adventure playground occupied only the southern border of this attractive old British garden which contained numerous mature trees, a central wide expanse of lawn, plus a variety of decorative plants bordering the stately 18th century stone mansion. The remainder still serves as the private garden of the owner, through whose generosity the adventure playground has been allowed to function since its origin in 1970.

The physical appearance of an adventure playground environment is normally constantly changing because its form and content is created by the actual users whose activities and interests are themselves continuously evolving. However, because of the relatively infrequent availability of this playground to most of the users, it contained a greater amount of permanently fixed equipment. This also served as a constant reference guide by which a child could orient himself. During this study, the adventure playground had 37 specifically identifiable activity areas, of which 14 qualified as being permanently fixed play structures.

These 14 fixed facilities consisted of a diverse assortment of custom-made forms and shapes intended to stimulate curiosity, novelty, adventure, muscular skills, self-confidence, and just plain fun. There was an 18-foot high climbing lookout tower with four platforms at varying levels. A simple pulley system suspended from the top railing allowed all kinds of equipment to be hauled up or lowered to friends below. The tower also served as the basis for the construction of many temporary structures built out from it such as additional steps, platforms and shelters. In the centre of the playground was a large jumping deck consisting of a 15-foot by 15-foot railed platform at 8 feet above ground, with a 5-foot by 5-foot opening in its centre through which a child could jump, slide, or simply fall on to the thick foam rubber pads below (Figure 7). This enabled even a blind child to safely experience the exhilaration of freely falling through space.

Two slides were incorporated with this platform - one leading directly to the ground while the other led to a free-fall ride through the platform opening. This structure, located on slightly elevated topography, also fulfilled an important function as a major focal point. Adjacent to the jumping deck was a concrete lined undulating free-form pond with depths varying from 4 to 18 inches. A choice of permanent and non-permanent bridges was provided to facilitate different ways of crossing to a large deep sand area on the opposite bank. At its widest point, the pond was used for 'boating' and all manner of innovative water play.

A short hose from a fountain allowed for the ever popular mixing of sand and water. Serving to unify the entire complex was a seven foot high overhead track structure which wound its way from the clubhouse to the high tower at the opposite end. A variety of apparatus could be suspended from this track to aid the mobility of children with ambulatory disabilities, i.e., wooden seat, canvas sling, etc. Since most of the ground surface consisted of plain loose earth, a continuous eight-foot wide tarmacadam path connected the entry gate to the clubhouse to provide a firm surface for the numerous wheeled vehicles, carts, scooters, wheelchairs, etc.

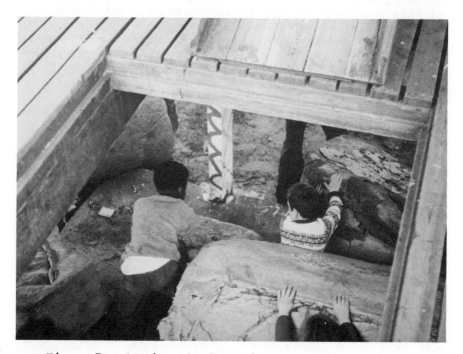

Figure 7: Jumping platform with foam rubber pads

The only other major permanent structure was a single storey 2,500 square foot clubhouse which contained a large central play space, an office, a kitchen, storage and toilet facilities. The central space was equipped with books, paper, paints, games and a wide assortment of toys primarily used in inclement weather. Juice for the children and coffee or tea for the adults were always available in the small busy kitchen.

The numerous less permanent facilities included two tents, a climbing cargo net, earth mounds of various heights, tire swings and climbing ropes suspended from the powerful branches of the shade-giving oak trees, a swinging and a rocking wooden plank, scattered large truck tires and tire ladders. Also on the site were an animal pen (rabbits and sick birds), a small vegetable garden, an ever-popular fire barbecue area, and even a favourite spot to dig for worms. Various types of mobile equipment were also available, including battery-driven or self-propelled cars, tricycles, wagons, hand pedalled tricycles, etc.

Except for some special provisions in the clubhouse and the overhead track structure, the physical facilities of the Chelsea adventure playground, though somewhat more compact and slightly more structured, basically differed very little from those of the other 86 adventure playgrounds now functioning in Greater London. And yet, this secluded half acre of activity on a Chelsea side street contained an environment and atmosphere so unique and rich as to defy adequate description. Although a similar playground is now being planned for the southern section of London, at the time of this study it was the only true adventure playground in existence anywhere, specifically designed and organized for the use of children with any kind of handicap, whether mental, physical or emotional, and in any degree of severity. Even though the playground remained closed on weekends, an average of 500 children per week made use of these facilities. The various schools which used the adventure playground included those for the mentally handicapped - such as the educationally subnormal (ESN) and mentally retarded; schools for the physically handicapped - spastic, spina bifida, partially sighted, blind, deaf and partially hearing; and schools for the emotionally disturbed, maladjusted and autistic. Most children were thus regularly exposed to others with similar or dissimilar handicaps.

In the literature on adventure playgrounds much justifiable emphasis has been given to the pivotal role of the play leader (Benjamin, 1966; Bengtsson, 1972; Lambert and Pearson, 1974). The title of play leader, however, seems to be a misleading one since his or her function is actually to guide and facilitate rather than to lead. A far more accurate term would appear to be that of play facilitator, or even play liberator. John Bertelsen, the first play facilitator of the original Danish adventure playground at Emdrup, 33 years ago, understood this position well when he stated:

"The children are sovereign and the initiative must come from them. The leader can make suggestions but must never demand. He must obtain the tools and materials needed or requested by the children but must at any time be prepared to give way to new activities. To organize and arrange programs is to stifle imagination and initiative and preclude children whose lively curiosity and interests constantly demand new outlets." (Lambert and Pearson, 1974)

Primarily through the sensitive and conscientious efforts of the young play facilitators of the Chelsea adventure playground, these special children are encouraged to explore the limits of their individual capabilities and initiative within the boundaries of safe practices.

COMPARISON OF BEHAVIOURS

Interpretation of these explorations must, of course, be tempered by two basic considerations. First, the small size of both subject groups limits the degree to which the findings can be generalized. Second, the start of the summer holidays and the consequent disbanding of the classes limited the length of time that the children were exposed to the two playgrounds. A longitudinal study of six to twelve months duration could provide valuable supplementary data by investigating the change and development over time relating to the play behaviour engaged in at each playground.

Observed behaviours

Within these limitations, however, the observations clearly indicated that the children displayed significantly dissimilar frequencies of behaviour at the two playgrounds (Figure 8).

	CONVENTIONAL PLAYGROUND		ADVENTURE PLAYGROUND	
	frequency	%	frequency	%
NON-SOCIAL				
solitary play	60	23.1	108	39.2
parallel play	133	51.2	21	7.6
SOCIAL				
positive inter-action with peers	36	13.8	140	50.7
positive inter-action with adults	31	11.9	7	2.5
	260	100%	276	100%

Figure 8:   Frequencies of behaviour for younger group at both playgrounds

The adventure playground stimulated a greater frequency of both the non-social behaviour of solitary play and the socially oriented behaviour of positive interaction with peers. The maximization of these two behavioural patterns is essential in providing the three most vital basic characteristics for optimal growth and development - independence (self-reliance) and initiative (self-motivation), both through solitary play; and active interest in the physical and social environment, through interaction with others (Norris, Spaulding and Brodie, 1957). Attainment of all three is particularly difficult for the blind and partially seeing. The appropriate play situation may well offer a primary context for their development.

While the relationship of social to non-social behaviour approached a ratio of 1:1 at the adventure playground, the conventional playground prompted a frequency of non-social behaviour that was nearly three times that of social behaviour. This was primarily due to the more frequent occurrence of parallel play at the conventional playground. The fact that the maximum behavioural frequencies were generated at different playgrounds suggests that these two play settings may be complementary rather than competing environments - each one being most appropriate in accommodating specific patterns of behaviour.

The results of a 1972 study by Bishop, Peterson and Michaels showing the preferences of non-handicapped eight year olds for various types of play equipment also suggests that adventure playgrounds may be "complementary to, rather than substituting for playgrounds that are primarily designed for physical activity". They found that the children differentiated strongly between the contrived - "designed for the purpose of play" - and uncontrived - "might be used for play but not intended for that purpose" - play environments. The latter comprised construction sites, junkyards and vacant lots while the former consisted of playgrounds offering conventional equipment mainly designed for physical activity (Bishop, Peterson and Michaels, 1972).

For the four and five year old visually handicapped, the two playgrounds are also differentiated by how they influence both the intensity and the change in intensity of play behaviour, depending on the length of time that the child is exposed to each setting. The frequencies of solitary play, parallel play and positive interaction with peers as condensed and averaged into a single 92-minute observation session, are illustrated in Figure 9.

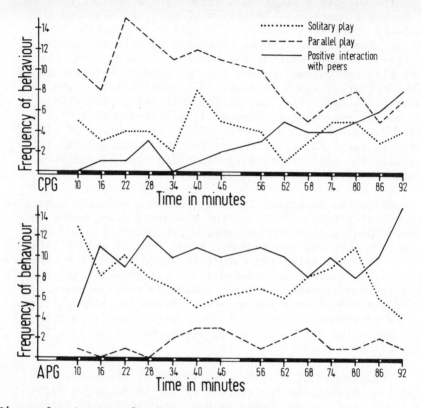

Figure 9: Average frequency of behaviour condensed to a
single play session

Despite the relatively short time scale, it appears
that extended exposure time is necessary at the conventional
playground to attain optimal levels of solitary play and
positive interactions with peers, whereas these levels are
experienced almost immediately at the adventure playground.
Also, if it were intended to maximize parallel play, the
conventional playground, particularly during the first hour,
would be the most appropriate setting. A considerably
longer period of participation would be necessary at the
adventure playground. This may be in part due to two related
factors. Firstly, the adventure playground may initially
be so stimulating that the child rapidly tries to sample as
many of the varied and novel stimuli as possible. This
involved mainly solitary play and positive interaction with
peers and very little parallel or imitative play. It should
be recalled that these children were only exposed to each

setting once a week. Therefore, the adventure playground
with its 37 diverse facilities may indeed be perceived by
the child as a novel environment at each visit.

The second factor is the opposite of over-stimulation,
namely, the repeated presentation of the same stimuli which
causes the 'orienting reaction' (Lynn, 1966) to become progressively weaker as habituation occurs. This would account
for the relatively low level of solitary play and positive
interaction with peers at the conventional playground, both
of which appear to require a diverse, novel and complex
environment. The bare asphalt school yard, which was the
play environment to which the children received the most
exposure, was totally devoid of any items that might sustain
an 'orientation reaction'.

Quantitative and qualitative aspects

Figure 10 clearly indicates that the quantitative
aspects of play for the younger children, as evidenced by
the number of changes of activity, has a discernably lower
frequency at the conventional playground than it has at the
adventure playground.

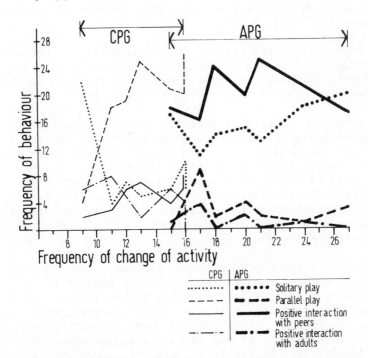

Figure 10: Frequency of behaviour related to changes of
activity at both playgrounds

The maximum number of changes of activity attained at the conventional playground is nearly coincident with the corresponding minimum promoted by the adventure playground. Except for the behaviour of one child who, because of more severe emotional problems, was subsequently transferred to a special school for the multi-handicapped, an increase in the number of changes of activity of the younger group promoted relatively little change in the constantly low frequency of solitary play at the conventional playground. This can be compared to a steady increase at a comparatively higher level for the adventure playground. The greatest frequency of all behavioural patterns at the conventional playground is evidenced by parallel play, which tends to increase slightly as a child engages in more changes of activity. At the adventure playground, however, parallel play has a very low frequency level and shows a marked decline in relation to an increase in the number of activity changes.

Positive interaction with peers and positive interaction with adults indicate a relatively low level of occurrence at the conventional playground, which is similar to that shown by solitary play. At the adventure playground the observed frequency of positive interaction with peers maintains a fairly constant high level while positive interaction with adults, on the other hand, remains at a constant and very low level.

Figure 11 is the result of combining all six behavioural categories to form the two classifications of social play and non-social play, and plotting them in relation to the frequency of changes of activity at both playgrounds.

Increased changes of activity shows a declining effect on social behaviour at the conventional playground and a consequent increasing effect on non-social behaviour; whereas it has comparatively little influence on the constantly high level of social and non-social behaviour which is reflected at the adventure playground. Even the highest level of social behaviour attained at the conventional playground does not reach the lowest level stimulated by the adventure playground.

Rank order correlation tests indicate that the same child who engaged in a greater number of changes of activity at the conventional playground also did so at the adventure playground. However, while that child's social behaviour at the conventional playground may have been relatively low, his social behaviour at the adventure playground, which was at a considerably higher level, was not appreciably affected.

There may conceivably be a certain frequency of changes of activity above which the frequency of social behaviour is no longer influenced.

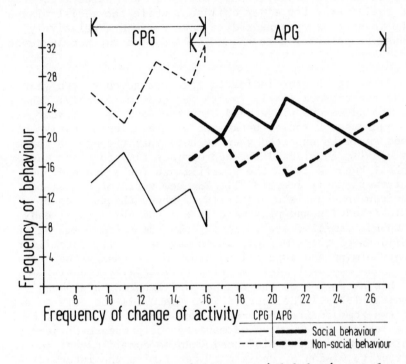

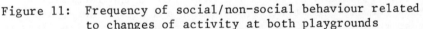

Figure 11:   Frequency of social/non-social behaviour related to changes of activity at both playgrounds

     Rank correlations further showed that an increase in changes of activity at the conventional playground corresponded to a greater frequency of positive interaction with peers, but did not relate to an increase of solitary play nor of positive interaction with adults. This suggests that positive interaction with peers, as well as parallel play at the conventional playground, can be increased by providing an environment that would stimulate more changes of activity while solitary play and positive interaction with adults might not be appreciably affected.

     The number and degree of variety of available facilities suggests one way of providing such an environment. The adventure playground contained over three and a half times the number of physical facilities that were provided at the conventional playground. As might be expected, a significant correlation existed between the number of available facilities and the frequency of changes of activity experienced in each playground.

For the older children, social behaviour and changes of activity at the adventure playground were highly correlated. Therefore, a greater number of changes of activity at the adventure playground related to a greater frequency of social play for older children, while the social play of the younger group appeared to have reached a relatively constant saturation level unaffected by a further increase in changes of activity.

The age factor indicated that the seven to ten year olds experienced nearly twenty per cent more social behaviour at the adventure playground than the four to five year olds. An increase of social behaviour with age during early childhood would be expected when we note that the age of three is usually considered the appropriate time to start nursery school because it is the starting age for sustained peer interactions (White, 1972). The new world of the school environment consists primarily of three things, two of which - adults and play materials - the child is already somewhat familiar with. It is only the third item, other children of the same age, which may be totally unfamiliar, overwhelming and even frightening to the young school starter. He may well seek security by initially focusing much of his attention on the teacher and ignoring his peers (White, 1972). The four to five year olds are only a year or two removed from this stage and could easily still be in the latter stages of adjustment to the presence of peers. This assumption is reinforced when we consider that the defective vision of these children limits the information they receive from their environment and from others, and that this tends to increase the initial time required for sustained social interaction (Huffman, 1957).

A desired optimal balance between social and non-social behaviour could conceivably be achieved by manipulating the environment to provide for the appropriate frequency of changes of activity. Since children with impaired vision commonly suffer from deprivation of adequate opportunity to communicate through social interaction, the most therapeutically beneficial play environment might be achieved by attempting to maximize the frequency of social behaviour as primarily represented by positive interaction with peers.

COMPARISON OF PLAYGROUNDS

How do these playgrounds differ in relation to their very dissimilar influences on the social and non-social behaviour of visually handicapped children? From the observational data and from extensive informal interviews in

both settings, these differences appear to consist of four
basic factors: the number of facilities, the type of facilities, the administrative structures and the adult role.

Number of facilities

Although the acreage of the two sites was very similar
(.43 and .45 acres), the number of physical facilities that
each contained was notably dissimilar. In a well documented
Building Research Station study of the play of normal children on 12 housing estates, Vere Hole (1967) demonstrated
that the acreage of an individual playground was not a major
determinant in its popularity. The number of facilities,
however, provided a much clearer basis of differentiation.
Although the conventional playground contained ten items,
the total number of different facilities was only seven.
At the adventure playground the number of physical stimuli
constantly varied due to the very nature of an adventure
playground, but because of the limited capabilities of its
users, this range (from 34 to 43 items) was much smaller
than is prevalent at most adventure playgrounds for the non-
handicapped. For the four to five year olds, the adventure
playground with 3.7 times the number of facilities of the
conventional playground is associated with 1.5 times as many
activity changes. Therefore, a single change of activity
is associated with nearly 2.4 times the number of facilities
at the adventure playground as compared to the conventional
playground. This suggests that although the large increase
in the number of facilities available at the adventure playground contributed to the increased frequency of activity
changes, it was not the dominant influence on this change
of behaviour.

Type of facilities

As previously noted, the equipment at the conventional
playground was of a fixed, static nature, giving a sense of
timeless permanence and oriented primarily toward physical
motor activity. All the equipment prescribed a specific
implied use with extremely little latitude for any choice
in behavioural response, i.e. slides, swings, roundabouts.
There was not the slightest suggestion nor illusion of the
user's ability to assert any change on the environment.

How do children generally respond when denied all
opportunity to cause an effect on their environment? At
many conventional playgrounds it is not difficult to find
swings, often the only movable items, that are twisted,

tied or greatly foreshortened by wrapping them around their top supporting member. This appears to reflect a vain and almost pathetic attempt to effect some change on a challengingly rigid environment. Frequently this motivation will result in a need for self-assertion through more destructive acts of vandalism. In the first major exploration of play behaviour, Groos, in 1901, recognized this basic need as the child's "joy in being a cause of a change to the environment" (Ellis, 1973).

The opportunity to be a "cause of change" is provided in many of the 14 fixed and 23 less permanent facilities of the adventure playground which are primarily of a flexible and dynamic nature. These objects form a strong contrast to the permanent galvanized steel structures of the conventional playground. Wood, either brightly coloured or left to reflect its natural patterns of grain and texture, is the dominant material. Although also providing for the development of large muscle skills, these facilities are oriented more towards direct involvement with the environment through exploration, manipulation and novelty. Whereas the equipment of the conventional playground was of such a nature as to confront the child with the implied question "what am I supposed to do with this" (i.e. climb up, sit or lie and slide down and then repeat), the facilities of the adventure playground promoted the questions "what do I want to do here" and "what am I able to do with this" (i.e. climb on it, in it, hide in it, pretend it is a fort, boat or castle, add to it, dig under it, etc.)

There is another distinct method of categorizing these two types of play facilities that could readily contribute to the behaviour provoked by each. In Piaget's penetrating questioning of seven and eight year olds, he clearly pinpoints the concept that this age group tends to equate 'life' to 'movement' (Piaget, 1929). A bicycle is considered 'alive' because it moves, so is a house, a cloud, the sun, the lake, a watch, and the wind; whereas a tree, a mountain or a table are perceived as devoid of life because they do not move. It is not inconceivable that this age group similarly categorizes some play environments as having life (movement) while others do not. Since many of the facilities at the adventure playgrounds were movable or facilitated movement (sand, tires, water, etc.), it is quite possible that this environment was perceived of as more 'alive' than the permanently fixed equipment of the conventional playground. It should be noted that Piaget defines four distinct stages in the development of the concept of life. In the first stage, life is attributed to everything that has

activity or a function of any kind. The second stage, as
described above, associates life with movement. During the
third stage, the child differentiates between movement which
is spontaneous (and therefore has life) and movement imposed
by an outside agent. In the fourth and final stage, life
is restricted to living organisms (plants and animals).
These concepts could be used to form the basis for further
investigation into the preferences for and images of different play environments by various age groups and how these
images would influence the child's physical and social
behaviour.

The administrative structure

The conventional playground which was located directly
across the street from the school, was a public city facility, although in practice it functioned as an extension of
the school environment subject to the authority and discipline of the school. Many rules and "don'ts" were still in
effect; (e.g. "don't climb on it that way, you may fall",
"don't run", "don't go down there backwards", etc.). Thus,
the children when taken out of their classrooms and into
the conventional playground experienced a welcome change of
surroundings but no basic change in administrative structure.

In contrast, the adventure playground was administered
by a private voluntary group known as the Handicapped
Adventure Playground Association (HAPA). Once the child
entered this setting, he was immediately under the responsibility of its staff which, it will be recalled, consisted
of a play leader and two or three assistants. Different
faces and voices and a wholly new administrative structure
was thus in operation, one which imposed only a minimum of
rules, e.g. "don't hurt others".

The adult role

In the conventional playground, the dominant adult
figure was the regular classroom teacher. The playground
itself was not staffed with any supervisory personnel or
play leaders. The activities of most of the four to five
year olds centred on the teacher's immediate vicinity, and
wherever she ventured her location became 'home base' for
all play. She had established a very good rapport with the
children and was in general well able to empathize with
their needs and frustrations, both in and out of the classroom. Yet, despite her sincere efforts, or possibly because
of them, much of the children's behaviour remained constantly

dependent on her participation. This is well illustrated by the relatively similar frequencies of solitary play and positive interaction with peers and adults.

The adult role at the adventure playground was manifested primarily by its invisibility, keeping within the concept of a true adventure playground. The play leaders, though always accessible, remained very much in the background. There was no adult-centred home base nor widespread dependence on adults for direction or guidance. The children appeared to perceive that this was their own territory in which there were few restraints, and they were free to sample and participate in any activity of their choice - or even to do nothing. And yet they understood that sympathetic adults were available to help with their special problems if and when they made the decision to seek their assistance.

The 30-minute bus ride from the school to the adventure playground provided an interesting minor study in contrasting behaviour. All along the route the school discipline was made to prevail within the tight confines of the minibus. The children were admonished to "sit still, stop yelling, no touching", etc. As soon as they arrived at the entrance to the adventure playground and the bus door swung open, all this suppressed energy was allowed to find free expression in an exuberant display of enthusiastic activity. This is clearly reflected in the high frequency of solitary play during the initial ten minutes of the play period.

The sudden reverse transition when the play session was concluded was considerably harder for both children and adults. Admonishments were more severe and much more frequent, with the teacher experiencing some difficulty in reasserting her authority. A week later, the identical cycle of joyful anticipation, exuberant release, active participation and reluctant recapture would be repeated. This entire sequence illustrates one of the major disadvantages encountered by restricting access to the adventure playground in such a way as to impose a seven day interval between visits. It should be recalled, however, that this unique playground was the only such facility available in all of London. Therefore, the large number of schools for all types of handicapped children who made use of this playground necessitated this restrictive policy.

FUTURE DIRECTIONS

Valuable information could be derived from longitudinal studies comparing the changes in social behaviour of handicapped children when exposed on a regular and frequent basis

to an adventure playground, conventional playground or to
no free-play environment at all. Of special interest may
be the fact that daily attendance at an adventure playground
would allow the child to engage in projects which could
continue over several play sessions, as in most adventure
playgrounds for normal children. This may affect the
creation of increasingly complex projects and a more personal
identification with specific items in the environment. It
may also result in greater social interaction and deeper
relationships among peers. An environment that can facilitate peer group interaction is not only beneficial to the
child's social development but also may relate directly to
his ability to perform physical tasks (Missiuro, 1963).
Further explorations of these factors could compare the
effects of various play environments containing different
quantities and types of peers, e.g. handicapped and non-
handicapped, on the child's ability to perform specific
motor activities.

The photographs serve to illustrate that the visually
handicapped were not the only ones using this playground.
Children with virtually all types of handicap were at various
times exposed to the facility. Thereby each child was
allowed to come in contact with peers possessing widely
divergent problems. The exploration of this unique situation
could significantly contribute to the continuing controversy
on integration versus segregation of the handicapped. The
Handicapped Adventure Playground Association is founded on
the premise that:

"The opportunity to go to specially designed and staffed
playgrounds where they can attempt and achieve all kinds of
physical and mental activities at their own speed and without the competition of more able children builds up in them
the confidence to venture into the more competitive world
outside." (HAPA, 1973).

Even if we accept this assumption (which has never been
objectively verified), it should be equally important to
compare the physical and social behaviour of those handicapped children exposed only to others with similar handicaps against those exposed to peers with widely differing
types of handicaps.

The adults concerned with these various groups were
unanimous in feeling that the adventure playground was a
very desirable and beneficial environment. Anyone who has
been exposed to this setting so full of love and understanding cannot help but concur. Most felt that in a pleasurable

way it challenged the children to use their maximum capabilities. Spastic and physically disabled children were seen to be motivated to use muscles that had long been considered inoperative. The mentally handicapped, who often found the adjustment from school to playground more difficult, were shown to be learning more from direct physical participation, e.g. lighting fires and discovering various ways of extinguishing them, than through other more formal teaching techniques. The maladjusted and emotionally disturbed were observed in more positive social interactions through involvement in cooperative projects with the physically and mentally handicapped. And the autistic, who exist in an often confused world of their own, quite divorced from reality, were seen to concentrate for extended periods on some particularly absorbing manipulative activity.

Although all of these positive behaviours were apparently associated with environmental influences, they are merely observations and qualified opinions, and still require validation through objective investigation. We understand extremely little of why they occur more frequently in certain settings. What specific factors in the environment help to promote these behavioural patterns? What factors tend to retard them? Clearly there is a great need to more fully comprehend the complex relationships between the play environment and its influence on social development, on the ability to engage in meaningful communications and on the content of the information that can be derived from it. We also need a far deeper understanding of those aspects of the environment which can help to increase the value of play "from which the child gains in knowledge through direct sensory experience, from which he enriches his spirit with the security of companionship and the discovery of beauty in his surroundings and from which he grows in stature and maturity by making demands on his vital organs, musculature and coordination." (Hutchins, 1970).

Over one hundred years ago, Friedrich Froebel was one of the first to recognize the importance of "freely chosen play". Yet the available choices within the child's world of home and school are highly structured and almost totally determined by others. It is only within the third world(!) of free-time activities that the child could readily be offered the freedom to explore, confront, challenge and experience according to his individual interests through participation in the creation of his own environment. Such exposure would allow the child itself to be a cause of change and thereby help to promote a feeling of effectance.

The great majority of play facilities are conceived, designed and executed as a total complete entity. Like most architectural edifices, once the first user occupies the facilities, they remain statically fixed. Although some alterations may be necessary from time to time, the need for such changes are rarely taken into consideration during the design process. The finished structure allows very little latitude for evolution. This inflexibility can severely restrict desired behavioural changes over time in most "functional" structures. Especially in play environments for the handicapped can it be totally self-defeating, since play motivation depends to a large extent on the arousal of curiosity, the opportunity for novelty and a "feeling of effectance" (White, 1972) through exploration, manipulation and social interaction.

The adventure playground is one of the few existing environments that is sufficiently adaptable and flexible to provide for this latitude of behavioural evolution. Its rate and direction of change are a direct result of the constantly changing behavioural patterns of its users. For the environmental designers these behavioural implications are still on the threshold of being recognized a major criteria for design equal to the standard factors of function, structures and beauty.

The visually handicapped child can readily be considered to form the extreme end of a continuum that encompasses all children from gifted to multi-handicapped. An environment such as the adventure playground that can be of therapeutic value to this child may indeed also be of significant benefit to other children. It encourages the child to explore, manipulate and fantasize. It can help to promote self-confidence by increasing interaction with others - especially with peers. It can be instrumental in increasing environmental awareness through participatory involvement. It can help the child to realize that he can effect a change upon the environment and thereby communicate something about himself.

ACKNOWLEDGEMENTS

I should like to express my sincere gratitude to the children of the John Aird School for the Partially Sighted in London, who, as the subjects of this study were also the inspiration for it. My thanks also extend to Mr. Bigness the school's headmaster, and to two dedicated teachers, Ms. Doral and Ms. Levickis.

For their joyful enthusiasm and cooperation, I also wish to thank the children of the numerous London schools and institutions for physical, mental and emotional handicaps, who participated in the Chelsea Adventure Playground programme, as well as its director, Ms. W. J. Pierce, M.C.S.P., and Paul Soames, its dedicated play leader.

I am especially grateful to Dr. David Canter, Director of the M.Sc. programme in Environmental Psychology at the University of Surrey, and George Miles, director of the London Centre on Environment for the Handicapped for their invaluable assistance and encouragement.

REFERENCES

BAYES, KENNETH and FRANCKLIN, S. (1971) Designing for the Handicapped, George Godwin, Ltd., London.

BENGTSSON, A. (1972) Adventure Playgrounds, Crosby Lockwood and Son, Ltd., London.

BENJAMIN, J. (1966) In Search of Adventure, National Council of Social Welfare, London.

BISHOP, PETERSON and MICHAELS (1972) Measurement of Children's Preferences for the Play Environment, EDRA 4.

BLOOM, B. S. (1964) Stability and Change in Human Characteristics, Wiley, London.

CHASE, R. A. (1973) Behavioural Biology and Environmental Design in Psychopathology: Contributions from the Social, Behavioural and Biological Sciences, Wiley and Company, New York.

DENNIS, W. et al (1957) "Infant Development Under Environmental Handicap", Psychology Monogram, 71 Whole N, 436.

ELLIS, M. J. (1973) Why People Play, Prentice-Hall, New Jersey.

FLAVELL, J. H. (1963) The Developmental Psychology of Jean Piaget, Van Nostrand, Princeton, New Jersey.

HANDICAPPED ADVENTURE PLAYGROUND ASSOCIATION (1973) Adventure Playgrounds for Handicapped Children, London.

HART, R. A. (1973) Environments for the Developing Child, Environment Design Research 4, Volume 2, W. Preiser (ed.) Dowden, Hutchinson and Ross, Stroudsburg, P.A.

HARTLEY, R. K. (1963) Verbalism among Blind Children, American Foundation for the Blind, New York.

HOLE, V. (1967) Children's Play on Housing Estates, Ministry of Technology, Building Research Station, Research Paper 39, H.M.S.O. London.

HUFFMAN, M. B. (1957) Fun Comes First for Blind Slow-Learners, C. C. Thomas, Illinois.

HURTWOOD, Lady Allen of, (1955) Planning for Play, Thames and Hudson, London.

HUTCHINS, H. C. (1970) Learning About Leisure in Relation to the Environment, Journal of Outdoor Education, Autumn.

JONES, B. (ed.) (1972) Ethological Studies of Child Behaviour, Cambridge University Press.

LAMBERT, J. and PEARSON, J. (1974) Adventure Playgrounds, Penguin, Middlesex, England.

LONDON ADVENTURE PLAYGROUND ASSOCIATION (1972) What is an Adventure Playground, N.P.F.A. London.

LOWENFELD, B. (ed.) (1973) The Visually Handicapped Child in School, John Day Co., New York.

LOWENFELD, M. (1967) Play in Childhood, John Wiley and Sons, New York, 1967.

MILLAR, S. (1968) The Psychology of Play, Pelican, Middlesex, England.

MISSIURO, W. (1963) "Studies on Developmental States of Children's Reflex Reactivity", Child Development, Vol.34, pp.33-41.

MOORE, R. (1974) "Patterns of Activity in Time and Space: The Ecology of a Neighbourhood Playground", in D. Canter and T. Lee (eds.) Psychology and the Built Environment, Architectural Press, London.

NORRIS, SPAULDING and BRODIE (1957) Blindness in Children, University of Chicago Press, Chicago, Illinois.

OAKESHOTT, E. (1973) The Child Under Stress, Priority Press, Ltd., London.

OPIE, I. and OPIE, P. (1969) Children's Games in Streets and Playgrounds, Oxford University Press.

PIAGET, J. (1973) The Child's Conception of the World, Routledge and Kegan Paul, London, reprinted by Paladin, London.

SCHOLL, G. T. (1973) Understanding and Meeting Developmental Needs in the Visually Handicapped Child in School, B. Lowenfeld (ed.), John Day Co., New York.

WHITE, R. W. (1972) The Enterprise of Living, Holt, Rinehart and Winston, Inc., New York.

WINNICOTT, D. W. (1971) Playing and Reality, Tavistock Publications, London.

WOLFF, P. M. (1975) Exploring the Influence of the Play Environment on the Social Behaviour of Visually Handicapped Children, unpublished Thesis, University of Surrey, Guildford.

WRIGHT, H. F. (1967) Recording and Analysing Children's Behaviour, Harper and Row, New York.

Physical Conditions and Management Practices for Mentally Retarded Children

SOFIA MAZIS AND DAVID CANTER

INTRODUCTION

Central to the concept of a therapeutic environment is the idea that there is some match between the physical form and content of the environment and the practices and organizational structure which are housed within the physical form. Although much of the discussion in the literature has been very general, there is a growing belief that the physical environment can play an active role in the therapeutic processes. Environmental psychologists such as Ittelson, Proshansky and Rivlin (1970), psychologists with a particular interest in mental retardation such as Gunzburg (1968, 1970, 1973, see the present volume), psychiatrists such as Osmond (1969, 1970), and architects such as Bayes (1967) all have presented arguments to suggest that the physical surroundings need to be examined whenever a therapeutic environment is being considered. However, although the significance of the physical surroundings has been recognized by a number of authors as a basis for empirical research, systematic studies which also incorporate an examination of the practices within the organization and the organizational structure are rare. Furthermore, the studies which have been carried out are generally within a very small number of rather specific settings and, as Ittelson (1974) and Canter (1974) in separate reviews point out, the studies which do exist may well have produced results which are idiosyncratic to the particular setting being studied.

The aim of the study reported here is to relate aspects of the physical environment directly to management practices and organizational structure. In doing this, an attempt is being made to see whether there are any patterns of relationship between the social processes of which an organization consists and the physical form in which it is housed. By exploring the nature of such a relationship we propose to open up for consideration the set of interrelated processes of which all aspects of the environment, physical, administrative and social, are a part. It is hoped that by doing this, two direct implications for practice will follow. First, that physical structures will not be provided in a way which is inappropriate for the organizational context in which those structures will be used. Secondly, that where an attempt is being made to modify the practices and experiences of building users, this will be done in the knowledge of the potential organizational relevance of physical designs, rather than in the naive hope that if a good 'design' is produced this will somehow generate good management practices and a good institution.

CONSIDERATION OF PHYSICAL VARIABLES

Although the study to be reported was concerned with institutions for mentally retarded children, it is appropriate to describe some of the physical variables which have been considered over the past 100 years or so as being of relevance to the design of therapeutic facilities. All of these variables have been identified as of significance for institutions for the mentally retarded but many of them were first or subsequently identified as being significant for a wide range of other therapeutic facilities.

(a) Size

As long ago as 1880 Kirkbride noted that there was an optimum size for an environment to be therapeutic. He was particularly concerned with facilities for mental patients. He made the point that there is a greater likelihood of patients losing their privacy and their identity amongst a large number of other patients, and further, the possibility for a friendly atmosphere being created was reduced as the institution increased in size.

This has been emphasized by many authors for almost all types of residential institutions. Kirkbride argued that the ideal number of beds in a hospital is 250 with an average of 15 patients on a ward. A number of mental hospitals were built based on these recommendations. However, the realization of the economic advantages and therapeutic efficiency in terms of specialized treatment led to the building of giant institutions, some of which have more than 2,000 patients. In the past two decades both the issue of economy and therapeutic efficiency with the large institution have come under strong attack. The emphasis has moved again to the small institution. Various recommended figures have been given. Haun (1950), Linn (1955) recommend hospitals with 250 to 400 beds. Baker et al (1959) suggest that hospitals should be no more than 300 beds in size with wards' of 30 beds. Patients should be grouped in 4 to 8 but progressing to larger groups of 10 to 15 as they improved. In relation to children the British Paediatrician Society (1962) recommended units with up to 60 beds and in 1971 the Department of Health recommended hospital units for children as being optimally of 24 beds.

There have been some studies (reviewed by Moos, 1974) relating size, amongst other variables, to the social environment within institutions. There have been very few studies examining the effect of size on the actual behaviour of patients such as the study of Wolfe (1975) on room size and behavioural patterns in a children's psychiatric hospital. Usually, however, the recommendations given are not the result of empirical research. They are typically rather vague and refer to personal experience of the experts making the recommendations, their beliefs about obtaining a balance between what is possible for management to organize efficiently, yet still maintaining a group of what is usually referred to as 'a family' size which will provide an effective level of social interaction. Inevitably where abstract ideas like social atmosphere are set in the balance against the seemingly more concrete issues of management efficiency, there is a tendency for the balance to swing towards the latter rather than the former. Hence the reason for the 'family' label being given to group sizes which would have been large families in Victorian days, let alone in the modern 4 to 6 person household.

(b) Layout

Layout of the hospital and of the beds within it have also frequently been considered. Certainly in post war years big compact buildings with long corridors have frequently been blamed for creating an institutional atmosphere which is counter therapeutic. Instead the 'villa' approach to hospital design has been advocated (Linn, 1955, for example) reflecting an earlier approach to hospital facilities. Baker et al (1959) tried to take this idea further and proposed a village hospital, where the social centres are located in a

focal position with the residential unit on the periphery.
Others such as Good et al (1965) even try to suggest that
the design could follow the rhythm of the therapy and propose
that spaces could be arranged in a continuum according to
the progressive changes in the treatment of a patient.
Osmond (1970) considered the social interaction of patients
as being more critical and proposed the notion of sociopetal as opposed to the more typical socio-fugal spaces.
This is a distinction which has crept into the popular
scientific literature, yet remarkably few researchers have
been able to demonstrate convincingly that the location of
any layout along this continuum, from socio-fugal to sociopetal, can be objectively measured.

Throughout all the literature the dominant discussion
does appear to be in favour of keeping groupings as small as
is manageable. The 1972 recommendations of the Department
of Education for schools and hospitals for severely handicapped children summarize these ideas as follows:

"The school as a whole can be seen as a series of bases
or group bases designed for the different needs of children
at each stage with other areas being available which are
common to all..."

The same document puts forward a more conventional architectural proposal which certainly has some intuitive appeal:

"The building should be flexible in use offering a
variety in size and character of enclosed spaces."

Yet as is so often the case in government documents
the terms such as 'flexibility', 'variety', and 'character'
are left to be defined by the creative imagination of the
design team. Indeed the design team can draw upon a caveat
which surely opens up the inventive opportunities produced
by the need for flexibility, variety and character, namely
that "spatial relationships should be simple so that children can readily understand the building".

As in so many other cases the discussion in the literature does little more than point to the need to consider
layout. It provides little detailed guidance on the way in
which layout may actually be handled beyond putting forward
concrete proposals as to how the authors themselves would
think of doing it with little evidence for why.

(c) Siting

The heritage of the placement of large asylums (for what were considered to be therapeutic reasons in the days that they were built) in remote rural areas, has been strongly criticized in more recent times. It seems to be increasingly believed that these facilities should be placed within the community and form an integral part of it. Authors such as Gunzburg (1973) and the Department of Education and Science (1972) provide practical reasons for such community based provision, such as easier staffing, better communications with visitors and helpers and more ready provision of day treatment facilities. It is also argued that the therapeutic processes are aided by providing patients with the opportunity to keep in touch with the normal life of the community. Certainly, placing facilities within a community must be distinguished from taking the therapeutic processes out into the community and little attention appears to have been given to the advantages of the large highly serviced institution as a basis for forays into the community. Little attention also appears to have been given to responding to the community reaction, or coping with the attitudes of those 'ordinary' people who may be less 'enlightened' than the policy makers.

(d) Interior atmosphere

Although consideration of the larger scale issues referred to above have occurred in the general literature on the creation of therapeutic environments, the majority of concern has been devoted to examining internal environmental issues. One reason for this is that the approach to therapy by 'milieu', which for years almost ignored the physical component, now takes the other extreme and readily fades into a concern for interior decoration, colour, shapes, materials, types of furniture and so on. Another reason for this is that this has been a very obvious area in which institutions have been lacking in the past, with their impersonal, monotonous decor. Further, the limited budgets under which most institutions are created, often leads to a reduction in the quality of design occurring late on in the design process when the most easy thing to reduce is the amount of money spent on fixtures and finishes.

The most enthusiastic supporters for the importance of the careful design of interiors within institutions are the Gunzburgs (1968, 1970, 1973), Bayes (1967) and Mesmin (1971). Much of the discussion of the interior environment focuses on the details, on the quality of small scale bits and pieces, aspects of decoration which are all too easily missed when small scale decisions are made by large scale organizations. The orientation here is towards (a) creating physical comfort and what is often referred to as "a sense of security of the surroundings", (b) producing a stimulating and interesting environment, which will respond to the capabilities of the users, and (c) providing the facilities for teaching and training relevant behaviour.

Such expectations of the physical surroundings are of course highly ambitious but are at least couched in a reasonably practical frame. However, it is not uncommon for authors to wax romantic. If not romantic then the emotional appeal implicit in the following quote from Bettelheim (1974) demonstrates the excesses of opinion which are possible.

"Designers of mental institutions should not rely on conveying meaning only through rational arrangements. They should also know that every detail of the building, action and attitudes is a carrier of symbolic meaning."

The recurrent theme in all this consideration of interior environment is the attempt to make these institutions more domestic or homelike. Almost all publications which relate to the design of institutions for mentally retarded children mention the need to attain a domestic character to the buildings. Yet it is rarely specified exactly how this should be achieved. The concern appears to be more to avoid the institutional character of many of the existing old buildings than to clearly create a particular type of environment. After all, there would be great differences in the design and use of the houses lived in by any set of people sitting round a table discussing the domestic character of a new institution. Some of the authors who have explored this issue more carefully, such as Baker et al (1959), have stated that it is not really possible to design in such a way that 30 people can be accommodated and to retain the atmosphere of a house for, say, five people in a family. Dwybad (1968) has also pointed to the possibility that by focusing on the 'home like' quality of an environment, a more significant goal of responding to the needs of individuals will be missed. According to Dwybad the challenge for the architect is "to create a new pattern to facilitate group living and yet provide space in which the individual can relate himself in a meaningful way". Behind this discussion is an emerging difference between two clearly identified schools of thought. One is epitomized by the concept of 'normalization'; (Nieje, 1970; Bank-Mikkelson, 1970) the attempt to create a setting which is as normal as is possible and thus creates the opportunity for the residents to move towards a more normal existence. The other school of thought is trying to put forward the argument (Dennis, 1965; Sandhu and Hendriks-Jansen, 1976) that the environment must be as stimulating as possible in order to provide some form of help to the residents whose cognitive and perceptual abilities will be much lower than normal. Nonetheless this distinction is not as great as it seems at first glance. The Gunzburgs (1973), for example, examining the concept of normalization, point out that a positive environment must be derived from the realization that the user is in some respects handicapped. Therefore he requires special support from the environment in order to help him live a comparatively active, normal life. Sandhu and Hendriks-Jansen on the other hand, are quite prepared to recognize that staff spend a great amount of time in these institutions and they must be taken into account as well in producing this 'stimulating' environment. Weeks (1972) has highlighted the key issues here:

"Often much is made of the need to avoid the atmosphere of an institution. In fact the characteristics of an institutional environment are not easy to describe, but perhaps one of the most important is that in an institution the control of the micro-environment is not that of the people for whom the institution is ostensibly designed. It is not particularly to do with size of rooms, scale of interior, presence or absence of carpets. It is whether the decisions about these things have been taken by the administration or the inhabitants. The essence of 'domestic' environment is that it is under the control of the inhabitants who arrange interiors according to the way they want."

What is being emphasized in this quotation is that the impact and significance of the environment cannot be clearly separated from the organization and administrative policies which are housed within it. It thus points to the fact that dealing with the physical variables as if they were isolated causal factors can lead to the confusions and ambiguities which have been referred to earlier. What is necessary is to explore the way in which the physical factors relate to organizational issues. The more academic question of why it would be expected that particular organizational forms would be found in particular physical settings may await empirical results before an answer is attempted.

ORGANIZATION AND MANAGEMENT PRACTICE

Besides the comments above pointing to the need to identify aspects of management practice in order to understand the relationship of the physical environment, it is instructive to consider Wittman's (1972) comment that:

"Drawing the relationship between physical space and therapeutic activities requires two kinds of information that are simply not available at the present time. A definite relationship...takes for granted the existence of a body of principles for treatment that would permit the derivation of propositions about the 'atmosphere' and social interaction that should be induced by the setting in order to maximize the therapeutic effects of the environment."

In other words it is necessary to specify the nature of the therapeutic processes which it is intended to house in order to understand the contribution which the housing makes to these processes. However, as many researchers have pointed out, it is extremely difficult to specify exactly what are the most effective therapeutic procedures. What does appear to be possible is to identify the general management practices which are commonly believed to be of value. However, even here caution must be exercised as Morris (1969) says with reference to mental subnormality hospitals:

"...we suggest that interpersonal relationships were at least as important as physical conditions in determining the kind of care given to patients. There is not necessarily any direct connection between the quality of nursing care or the educational and training facilities and the decrepitude and unsuitability of many of the buildings, although the relationship needs to be investigated systematically."

However, having identified the quality of care, social organization, organizational structure, or whatever of the labels are used for describing the activities and practices which make up the institution, there is the much more difficult step of measuring in some reasonably objective way the social and behavioural aspects of institutions. The literature which exists tends, on the one hand, to be cast in the case study mould such as the classical study by Stanton and Swartz (1954) who produced a complete picture of the human relations within a mental hospital. There are a few comparative studies such as that of Wing and Brown (1970) but they are still descriptive of a number of cases. On the other hand, institutional settings of the sort with which we are concerned occupy a very small part of the

general literature on organizations and are generally regarded by organizational theorists (e.g. Blau and Scott, 1963,
or Etzioni, 1961) as a quite distinct category of organizational type. Indeed, it is even difficult to establish a
precise definition of exactly what a residential institution
is because so little attention has been given to it by
organizational theorists. Rather the attempt has been made
to distinguish residential institutions from other sorts of
organizations. Parsons (1960) for example has pointed out
that institutions can be distinguished from other organizations by the fact that they take the customer into the
organization.

"In these organizations the recipient of the service
becomes an operating member of the service."

Goffman, in his classic work on asylums (1961), really
extended Parsons' idea to highlight the fact that certain
residential institutions may be regarded as 'total institutions'. Goffman characterized total institutions as places
in which (a) the people living in them conduct all aspects
of their life in the same place and under the same single
authority, (b) each aspect of the residents' daily activity
is carried out in the immediate company of a large group of
others, and (c) all phases of the day's activities are
tightly scheduled, the whole sequence of activities being
imposed from above by a system of explicit formal rules.
It can be seen that the most obvious example of a total
institution is the prison. It was in pointing to the fact
that a number of other institutions, notably those which
were explicitly intended for therapeutic purposes, had many
similar characteristics to prisons, that gave such weight
to the argument that many institutions were not achieving
the therapeutic goals set for them.

It was by identifying the characteristics of total
institutions that Goffman laid clear the path for a more
systematic examination of the activities of which the institutions consist. By exploring carefully the issues to which
Goffman had drawn attention and putting this together with
the general agreement that a move away from the institutional
qualities of total institutions towards more domestic qualities was a commonly agreed goal to be struggled for, it
became possible for researchers to develop techniques for
assessing the organizational nature of residential institutions. King, Raynes and Tizard (1971) were the most notable
researchers in developing a set of scales to measure the
ways in which institutions operate. The fact that their
scale was developed for handicapped children makes it

particularly appropriate to our current concern. They were
able to demonstrate that there are large differences in the
everyday life of institutions which were significant for
the residents of those institutions yet could be identified
from the way in which staff behaved towards the residents
in daily activities and routines. We will return to the
scales and the developments later, but now we must consider
the particular setting and institutions studied here.

RESIDENTIAL INSTITUTIONS FOR MENTALLY RETARDED CHILDREN

Exact figures on the prevalence of subnormality do not
exist and precise estimates are difficult to obtain. However, according to the Department of Health and Social
Security (1971) there are probably about 120,000 in England
and Wales who are severely mentally handicapped, of whom
about 50,000 are children. Many more are mildly mentally
handicapped.

The care of subnormal people has taken many forms.
When the National Health Service started in 1948 the responsibility was transferred from local authorities to the new
hospital authorities. Major changes took place again in
1959 when the Mental Health Act was published. The Royal
Commission which examined the issue put emphasis on community
care and on the end of segregation, and laid the duty on
the local authorities to provide a full range of community
services including residential accommodation for the mentally
retarded. More recently in 1971, local authorities became
responsible also for the education of mentally retarded
children, who up until that time were excluded from the
educational system. Against this background of a hetero-
genuous group with a wide range of definitions and a variety
of changes of organization which have taken place in Britain
in the past thirty years, it is not surprising that there
are a great variety of institutions for mentally retarded
children. There are, for example, units within hospitals,
junior training centres, hostels and a host of other possibilities. Indeed, many officials at central government
and local government level encourage the development of
alternatives as a way of testing the various possibilities
available. The most common forms of institution are subnormality hospitals and special schools. These institutions
provide residential accommodation for a large number of
children who, for various reasons, cannot be kept with their
families. The attempt is made within these hospitals and
schools, besides providing medical treatment and education,
to prepare the children for future employment and to enable
them to look after themselves as independently as possible.

For the present study it was decided to concentrate on those institutions which most closely reflected the form referred to as a total institution. This covered institutions which officially are referred to as children's units in mental subnormality hospitals and also boarding schools for mentally retarded children. It excluded, for example, hostels or children's homes, in which the children may only eat and sleep and go from there to some other institution for their education. A further criterion was used in order to eliminate other possible organizational influences. This was that the institution should be under state control, in the sense that they are maintained or registered with the local authorities and are not privately financed or administrated. One further practical criterion for selection must be mentioned. They were all to be within a day's commuting distance of the researcher's base. This practical consideration led to the selection of institutions situated in part of South East and South West England.

Institutions were selected from the Department of Education and Science 1974 list of "Special Schools for Handicapped Children in England and Wales". A letter was sent to the head of a total of 63 establishments, selected from this list. Thirty-seven replies were received and of these a great majority were very welcoming and friendly. From these replies it was possible to make visits to twenty of the institutions. These twenty provided the data base for this study.

The visit consisted of a day at the institution. During this time it was possible to obtain information on the child management practices within the institution and to be shown over it in such a way that notes could be made about its physical organization and structure. In some cases it was necessary and possible to talk to a number of members of staff in order to obtain all the information on child management. In other cases a well informed, loquacious informant provided all the detail that was necessary and considerably more besides. It is worth noting that although only twenty days of visits were involved, considerably more time was necessary to deal with the administration of the project. When the total amount of time and effort involved is taken into account, it comes as no surprise that most researchers have only the resources to deal with far fewer institutions.

Furthermore, a great variety of buildings existed even in this supposedly homogeneous organizational sample. Apart from their varying ages, a variety of previous uses as well as recent changes and additions were apparent across the sample. Some were housed in 16th century manor houses whilst others were in new specially designed accommodation with most combinations between.

The child management scale

By extensive observations in a large number of institutions King, Raynes and Tizard found considerable differences in various aspects of what they called "child management patterns". From these observations they were able to classify institutions along a dimension running from those which had a "child oriented" pattern of management to those which had an institution oriented pattern of management. In the former the child is treated as a person rather than a number and there is less social distance between the children and the staff. The latter type of institution is characterized by rigid and restricted organization of a child's life. They developed a set of scales consisting of thirty items divided into four categories, each dealing with an aspect of management. These scale items enable them to give a total "child-management" (C.M.S.) score as well as scores under each of the headings of "rigidity of routine", "block treatment", "depersonalization" and "social distance". The full set of thirty items is given in Appendix A.

By relating these scores to other organizational variables they were able to find some of the correlates of child management patterns. Briefly they found: (a) that differences in child management patterns are not related to the kinds and degrees of handicaps of the resident children, (b) that they are not related to the overall size as measured by the number of children in an establishment, (c) that they are not related to the designated staff/children ratio within the institution but they are related to the effective staff/children ratio and (d), the most important organizational characteristic which relates to child orientation is the distribution of roles of the staff and the responsibilities of the head of the unit. They summarized the conclusions of their study by pointing to the fact that those units which were at the child oriented end of the continuum tended to have an organizational form which is akin to that of a household.

Clearly many of the items on their scales might be expected to relate to the physical provisions available. Take for example question 20, whether there are pictures, pin-ups or photographs in rooms. This, together with staff's attitudes on this issue, could readily be a function of the finishes and materials used within the rooms as well as the layout of the spaces within them. Many of the other questions could be examined in the same way. However, of central interest is that the scale has been related to "household organization". This accords well with the general design literature reviewed earlier, which stresses the advantages of producing 'domestic' facilities. By relating the two perspectives together it should be possible to clarify the nature of the physical facilities which may be regarded as domestic and whether they do indeed relate to child centred management practices.

One further advantage of using a standard scale is that it allows comparison between the present study and earlier ones and thus allows a test of generalizability of the results. King et al explored a wide range of institutions and obtained a mean for subnormality hospitals on their overall scale of 22.6. For the current set of twenty residential institutions the mean score was 22.5. This indicates general comparability between the institutions studied here and those studied by King et al.

Child management practice and organizational variables

The present study made it possible to examine the striking finding of King et al that child management patterns were not related to organizational size. Most students of organizations would agree with Blau's 1956 opinion that "While large size makes specialization possible and necessary, it also leads to a hierarchy of authority, a system of rules and impersonality". Commenting directly on institutional settings Ittelson (1974) points out that "Size of institutions is seemingly a critical factor, out of sheer administrative necessity the large institutions often find it necessary to regiment inmates to an extent which the small institutions consider undesirable".

The present set of twenty institutions covered a broad range of sizes and therefore correlation between the number of children in the institution and the child management score was of some interest. Its value was -0.1. This was closely similar to King et al's results supporting the general trend they found. However, experience of the institutions led to a questioning of whether the number of children housed was an appropriate index of organizational size. The organizational psychology literature, as well as the ecology literature (notably Barker and Gump, 1964), is concerned with the total size of an institution not with the number of people in any major component group. A correlation was therefore calculated in which the 'size' of the institution was taken as the size of the overall unit of which the children's institution was a part. Where it was part of a hospital the size of the hospital was taken as

the figure. Where it was an autonomous unit the size of
that unit was used. Using these figures the correlation
between size and overall child management score was 0.61.
This is a clearly significant correlation and so demonstrates
that this organizational variable does have implications
for child management practices. However, it must be remembered that the size here is confounded with organizational
form, because the larger organizations were those which were
hospital based. It would therefore appear to be the case
that it is not size itself which is the dominant correlate
but some aspect of organizational structure which size reflects.

Staffing

Because of the clearly critical value of the staff/child
ratio in an institution, this variable was also considered.
Some researchers such as Tizard et al (1972) have found that
children in institutions with better staffing show better
language development, and Ullman (1967) that the number of
staff per patient in mental hospitals is significantly correlated with the length of patient hospitalization. Further,
King et al had found that the higher the 'effective' staff/
child ratio the more child oriented was the pattern of
management likely to be. Unfortunately in the present case
it was not possible to calculate an effective staff/child
ratio (i.e. the number of staff on duty at the peak hours
of the daily routine). It was only possible to ascertain
the number of people who were available to take care of the
children. This number included both senior and domestic
staff as well as full-time and part-time staff. This did
not show any significant relationship with the child management scale. However, the average ratio was one member of
staff per 2.24 children and it only ranged between 1 to 1
and 1 to 3.6. It is therefore possible that the homogeneity
of staffing ratios was too great to reveal any relationship
to the management scale.

Organizational form

It is now necessary to turn to more qualitative aspects
of the organization. There was a large variation between
the different institutions in the way they were organized
and structured. In order to impose some pattern on this
range two broad categories of institution or organization
were identified, the second category being divided into two
sub-groups.

Group 1

Group 1 consists of children's units in mental subnormality hospitals. This accounted for nine of the twenty
institutions studied. The size tended to be around 70 children, but the size of the hospital to which they belonged
varied between that for 120 adults and children and one for
1,100 adults and children.

Because of their membership of the hospital these institutions have many characteristics in common with each
other, being a quite homogeneous group. None of them are
autonomous organizations but all are treated as an integral
part of the hospital of which they are a part. Further, the
life of the children is related to two authorities, the
Department of Health and Social Security which has the overall responsibility for the residential life and treatment
of the children, and the Department of Education and Science
which has responsibility for their education. It is curious
that visits indicated that both formally and informally
there is little co-operation between the two authorities
which have responsibility for the same children at the same
place, and sometimes even within the same building in that
place. Indeed, at times the impression was gained that
each organization tried desperately to keep its boundaries
strictly demarcated. It should be noted that this is not
an abnormal division, in that the child living at home also
experiences the split between his home environment and his
school environment, but not all parents agree that this is
necessarily a good thing. A further curious aspect of this
split, which was apparent from visits, was that the wards
in which the children slept tended to have a more clinical
and regimented atmosphere than did the schools. This is an
antithesis to what might be found in a conventional comparison of home and school. Indeed, at times the impression
was gained that the school was something of a relief from
the hospitalization within the residential accommodation.

The child management scale indicated that as a group
these institutions had a management pattern focused at the
institution oriented pole of the continuum. There was also
relatively little variation in the child management scores,
yet a great difference in the mean scores of this category
compared with the other two.

Group 2

This category consists of the autonomous institutions
which are officially referred to as boarding schools for

mentally retarded children. They are all under the authority
of the Department of Education and Science. Two structural
differences within this group can be identified to generate
two sub categories.

(a) Five of the twenty institutions studied fell into this
category. This tended to be the bigger of the two sub groups
(with an average size of 96 children). Their main characteristic is that each was one organization, with one individual
headmaster or headmistress having the overall responsibility
for its functioning. This one individual, in general terms,
is responsible for all activities both residential and educational in which the children are involved. The staff under
him, although being divided clearly into senior and domestic
staff, nonetheless have less distinct roles than in the category 1 institutions. Resident teachers, for example, may
be involved as play leaders with the children or with looking
after them in their residential activities.

Whilst on average they tend to show a child oriented
pattern, the distribution of scores is very great. This
would point to the dominant role of the head of the institution who can set in motion very different patterns of activities.

(b) A further six institutions may be characterized by being
registered with the local authority rather than being maintained by it. In other words although they are under the
responsibility in a general sense of the Department of
Education and Science, they are less directly supervised
and dependent upon this external agent. They were usually
founded by, and frequently to some extent funded by, private
organizations. Thus they had more freedom to develop in
ways which they consider appropriate. This freedom has led
all but one of these institutions to be sub-divided into
smaller 'family' groups containing between eight and sixteen
children. Thus there is no one individual who has total
responsibility in the same sense that a headmaster does in
category (a). This is because house parents are clearly
identified and are given some degree of real autonomy in
their activities.

As such these organizations correspond to what King et
al call "the household organization". It is not surprising
that, as a group, these institutions had a child management
score which was considerably lower than the other two categories.

Assessing the physical environment

As was pointed out earlier, there is little definitive, specific information available on the aspects of the physical environment which should be provided. Terms such as 'flexible' or 'having a human scale' or even 'homelike' have a great many ambiguities associated with them. In order to proceed further it was therefore necessary to identify clearly some aspects of the physical environment which could be recorded and which might be expected to relate to the other issues with which we are concerned. Ten such aspects were identified by placing an architectural interpretation upon the literature. They are presented here for general consideration in the hope that others may be able to refine and develop them.

1. 'Within the community'

This was taken in its simplest form to mean that an institution should be situated within a residential area or within less than thirty minutes walking distance of a village or neighbourhood centre.

There was some difficulty in assigning a score to a hospital, in particular, on this item. They all had extensive grounds and in many ways formed their own separate neighbourhood, even in the cases where they were located within a high density residential area. As a consequence, only one of the hospital units received a positive score. This was one with a small annexe situated within a residential area. Of the remaining twelve institutions, two are in remote rural areas with no access at all, two are in rural areas but are approximately six miles from small villages. One is near a village but cut off from it because of woods and a busy motorway.

2. 'Division into smaller units or living units'

This follows the recommendation by the DHSS (1972) that buildings should be divided up into physically separated and self-contained units and that they should not be designed for more than 24 children. Of the institutions visited, three belong to the 'corridor type hospital' and of a further six all activities were housed in one large building. Five other institutions were housed in 'villa type' settings and therefore typically were divided into living units. A further four were built in the form of cottages, each cottage including sleeping areas, living rooms, kitchen and staff rooms. One was so small, containing twelve children, that it is its own living unit. One further case was interesting in that although it was a large compact building it had recently been converted into living units, rather akin to conversion to a block of conventional flats.

3. 'Small sleeping spaces'

Although there is no standard number of beds recommended in the literature the emphasis is upon small bedrooms instead of large dormitories. It was found that institutions divided quite readily into those which contained bedrooms with up to eight beds and those with dormitories with approximately twenty beds. The first group were therefore taken as positive and the second group as negative. Occasionally these larger dormitories did have one or two small side rooms for disturbed or temporarily sick children. Two hospitals did have the dormitories divided up into two rooms with a night nurses' station in between. For those ten institutions with eight or less beds, five have a mixture of room sizes with three to eight beds and five had bedrooms for four children each. This range of sizes alone raises many questions as to what exactly the logic is at the present time for providing any particular one.

4. 'Proximity of the kitchen'

A number of authors, notably Gunzburg (1970) and Rivlin (1972) have pointed to the significance of the kitchen in an institutional setting. Certainly in any domestic setting the kitchen would be found to be an important place where the child interacts with adults and learns about many of the things upon which domestic survival is based. In many institutional contexts as well, the kitchen is often a stimulating and interesting place in which to be. It was therefore considered that, contrary to the management convenience and possibly the economy of central isolated kitchens, open and physically accessible kitchens serving a specific unit were to be preferred. For our purposes a positive score was given to an institution in which the kitchen was in the same building and on the same floor (because of children in wheelchairs) as those spaces in which most of the domestic activities of the children were carried out. This was usually the day room and so it was simply a matter of noting whether the kitchen was in the same building and on the same floor as the day room.

Again, eight of the hospitals fell into the group which did not have readily accessible kitchens. Meals were carried by trolley and served either in a communal dining room or

in a sitting room of the villas. For some peculiar reason
one institution had the kitchen located in the administrative
building and meals were served in yet another block. Seven
of the more compact buildings had the kitchen on the ground
floor, usually visible and inter-connected with the ground
floor dining room. Three of the institutions built in the
cottage system had a kitchen in each cottage with the meals
being cooked for the particular group living in that cottage.
As in a private home the kitchen tended to be used for a
whole range of other informal activities in these places.
Finally, in one small building the kitchen was designed to
be part of the living room making an open plan kitchen-
dining room.

5. 'Adequate toilet facilities'

The idea of including this item emerged during visits
to the institutions. It became obvious that people working
in the various institutions put great store on the design
of sanitary facilities. Surprisingly, however, it was difficult to find any standards or precise guidelines in the
literature except for some general statements about the
number of toilets per person. No mention was found of the
distribution of toilets, nor their size and particular location within the building. In order to get a general index
it was decided to take the staff reactions into account and
therefore a positive score was given to any institution
where no complaints about the toilet facilities were made.
Seven of the institutions had serious problems with the
toilets. In one, for example, there was complete lack of
bathing facilities and separate staff toilets. In two other
institutions children, or staff carrying children, had to
cross all the classrooms in order to visit the toilets. In
another two institutions they had to walk some distance to
get to the separate sanitary accommodation. In one the
toilets were in a draughty corridor open on both sides to
the weather. In possibly the worst case, the toilets were
so old and decayed that it was difficult to see what could
be done to make them any less filthy.

Of the remaining thirteen institutions there was a
further one which obtained a negative score because the head
of the institution reported that they did not need a group
of toilets, but a number of smaller units for each group of
children to facilitate the work of the staff. Nonetheless
in the twelve institutions to which a positive score was
given there was still comment about the lack of surfaces on
which children could be placed and changed by the staff.
Indeed, only one new, purpose built, building had all the
necessary provision and the staff were extremely pleased with
this.

6. 'Privacy'

Under this heading we put a number of small details of the institutions which enables the children to have some privacy. Official publications such as the DHSS (1971) report refer to the need for such facilities to be present. On this basis a positive score was given to an institution in which the following were provided: curtains in the windows, partitions between the beds and doors on the toilets and bathrooms.

In going round institutions it was found that a common difficulty was that privacy for the children provided obstructions for easy supervision by the staff. There was furthermore a fairly common attitude that children and particularly mentally retarded children, do not need privacy. As a consequence it is not surprising that in fifteen institutions visited no provisions had been made for the children's privacy apart from curtains on the windows. In a few there were not even doors on the toilets. However, in five institutions various aspects of privacy have been provided for, most particularly the children have been provided with their own corners constructed either with movable partitions or cupboards.

7. 'Interior Quality'

As has been referred to earlier, there is frequent reference in the literature to the need for a stimulating and homelike environment. For our purposes it was possible to distinguish between institutions which had a monotonous institutional environment and those where vivid colours, differentiation of decoration from one space to another and the use of attractive materials together with non-standard equipment, pictures and personal belongings, were in evidence. These latter institutions were given a positive score.

In general it was found that the staff and authorities have tried their best to maintain a good standard and to produce pleasant surroundings as far as financial considerations and the building structure would allow. Only one out of the twenty institutions showed a neglect of this aspect, having monochromatic and empty rooms. Ten of the institutions presented a very high quality of interior design, having such items as carpets, individually selected equipment and even in some cases wooden panelling and fine old furniture. There were indeed two institutions in purpose built buildings, which had used expensive materials and careful design to the extent that 'luxurious' would be an appropriate adjective to describe them.

8. 'Controllable environmental elements'

The general point here is whether provision was made for the children to be able to modify the environment themselves. A simple example of this is that the heights and designs of door handles are such that at least older children can open them. Also the provision of light switches being accessible to children and lighting and heating being available for their individual rooms, in such a way that the children themselves can modify them. Surprisingly, although a matter on which many people would comment in their own homes, this is not something widely discussed in the literature. However, it did seem to be a simple indication of whether the environment had really been designed to cater for the children or the staff. A further point is clearly demonstrated here in that the attitudes of the institutions towards the children, on whether they should be allowed to control their own environment in some simple way, could be readily reflected in small design details.

Of those institutions visited, eleven held the positive view that the children should be able to use facilities and modify aspects of their environment as far as possible. Specially designed and even double door handles on the doors, as well as specially designed taps, had been put into these settings. All these institutions had also introduced ramps for children with wheelchairs. However, nine of the institutions had the opposite attitude. Changes had in fact been made so that children could not reach switches or open windows or even reach the bolts on the doors. This was usually considered to be necessary for the safety of the children.

9. 'Good maintenance'

This really covers the overall impression of the state of decorative repair and cleanliness of the buildings. The notable point that emerged under this heading, when visiting institutions, was that almost all of them were very clean and well maintained. Staff reported that all the rooms were decorated routinely every one or two years. It was even apparent in some institutions that cleanliness was considered the most important environmental aspect to achieve. Only five institutions did not achieve a positive score on this criterion. Of these two were housed in such an old and unsuitable building that it was difficult to maintain the buildings well. One was in a state of some disrepair because of building work, which was in progress. A further two were not well maintained and in need of some repair, the staff reporting that they did not remember the last time the building had been decorated.

10. 'Improvements'

This last item is taken from Morris's 1969 "Environment Index". The essence of this was to give a positive score to those institutions in which some things in the environment had actually been made by the children themselves. This usually involved the staff helping the children to decorate their rooms, make items of equipment or introduce other building modifications.

In eleven of the institutions it seems that no effort had taken place at all by the people who live and work within them to improve them. In three of these the attitude seemed to be that what they needed was a new building and that nothing could be usefully done with the existing one. The opposite side of this coin was shown in two institutions which had new buildings and here the staff admired what had been done for them and tried to keep it as it was. In the remaining nine institutions it appeared that things were being made continuously and often were regarded as having some educational scope. In two of the institutions the heads had taken a very special interest in having the children create innovative and interesting modifications, almost using the building as an educational toy.

The environment score

In order to obtain some overall score on the environment a scale score was calculated in such a way that if the institution was positive on a particular item it achieved a score of 1. These scores were then added together to give a total scale score for that institution. In other words this procedure gave each institution an 'environment' score which varied from 0 to 10. Clearly this is an attempt to develop some simple form of cumulative scale. The numbers of examples is not really great enough to test the scaleability of these items effectively. However, calculations which were carried out did indicate that these ten items related reasonably well to each other and could for the purposes of this exploratory exercise be regarded as a cumulative scale. Clearly much more work is necessary in the development of these items to turn them into a standard scale. For the present time, they are simply presented as a first approximation of the general environmental state of the institutions which facilitates comparisons for child management practices.

However, there is an interesting point about a scale of this type, should it be effectively developed. Unlike most standard psychological scales, one such as this, based upon statements about the physical state of the building, can be, in a sense, turned upon its head and used as a prescriptive guideline for design decision making. In other words, a designer or manager of an institution can check through the scale, once it is validated, and see where his own institution falls short and can then use this as very specific guidance for future action. We shall turn to this point in the conclusion.

RELATING ENVIRONMENTAL CONDITIONS
TO CHILD MANAGEMENT PRACTICES

Having calculated a child management score for each of the twenty institutions and an environment score for each of these institutions as well, it is a simple task to compare the ranking of the institutions on each of these measures. Figure 1 shows the relationships. It can be seen that this is a remarkably neat pattern, showing a clear tendency for the low child management scores, i.e. institutions which are child oriented, to have high environment scores, i.e. a pleasant or 'good' physical environment. The Spearman's rank order correlation of these scores gives the rather impressive figure of 0.92. Taking each of the sub divisions of the child management scale produces the following correlations: rigidity of routine correlates 0.95, block treatment 0.93, depersonalization 0.89 and social distance 0.94. There is thus very strong evidence that there is a close relationship between general aspects of the environmental design and a wide range of aspects of child management practices.

However it will be remembered that there were three distinct categories of institutions. It is quite possible that the overall structure of the institution is such that this has had a dominant influence on these scores, so adding little to our understanding of the relationship between child management practices and the physical environment. It was felt that this matter needed to be explored further although the numbers are rather small. To do this, the relationships between child management practices and the environment score were looked at within each of the three categories. This is illustrated in Figure 2. For Group (2a) there is a perfect correlation of 1.0 between child management score and environment score. The correlation is still statistically significant at 0.61 for Group (1), but it fails just to reach significance for Group (2b), being 0.56. This set of relationships clearly has something to

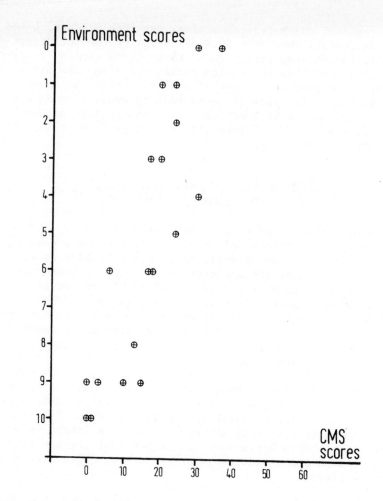

Figure 1: Relation between child management scores and 'environment' scores

do with the heterogeneity within each of the groups as Group (2a) is clearly the most heterogeneous group. Furthermore, Group (2b) does so well in comparison that some type of range effect is quite likely to be occurring, in that all the institutions are so relatively good that there is little real possibility of finding differences between them with instruments as crude as the ones we have been using. Of particular interest is the correlation for Group (1). This does show that although the institutions are all part of one large, centrally controlled authority, there is a great variety between them. As a consequence there is considerable room for improvement for those which are so poor in comparison with the rest of their group. However, it does

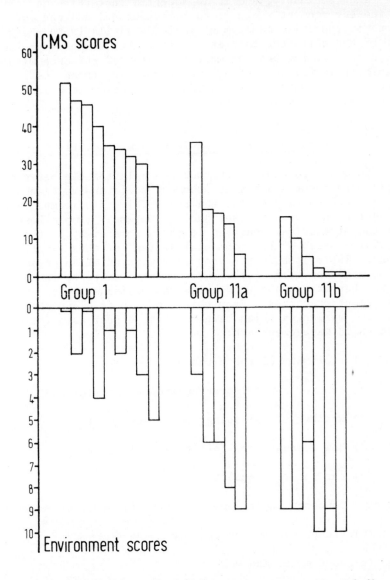

Figure 2: Distribution of child management scores and the 'environment' scores in the three groups of institutions

demonstrate that as a group those in category (1) have a great deal which they can learn from those in category (2b). There is no overlap at all between these two groups. The best of category (1) is still worse than the worst of category (2b), both on the child management scale and on the environmental scale.

If the value judgments implicit in the statements above are taken seriously, and it is accepted that the high score on the environment scale is to be encouraged and the low score on the child management scale is similarly to the benefit of the children, then it is clear that the present location of institutions for mentally retarded children within hospitals is far less effective than giving these institutions some autonomy of their own, in relation to a more local and focused authority.

Relation to specific environmental variables

In order to explore further the relationship between child management and the environment scale analyses were carried out on each of the environmental scale items. Again a caution must be expressed due to the small sample here, but the statistical analyses do throw some light on the crucial aspects of environmental design for these institutions. Table 1 shows the frequency with which an organization achieved each of the environmental factors, in relation to whether it was above or below the median score on child management practices. From this table it is clear that the physical variables which have the most direct association with child management are:

(a) proximity of the kitchen

(b) ease of control over environmental elements

(c) whether the sleeping spaces are small

(d) how adequate the toilet facilities are

(e) the interior quality

and at a somewhat lower level of statistical significance:

(f) the provision for privacy

(g) good maintenance

It is interesting to note that location within the community, the improvements and the division of the living units, do not relate at all closely to the child management scale. On the other hand, it is worthy of considerable attention that the proximity of the kitchen and the control over environmental elements have an almost perfect relationship with child management practices.

Table 1: Association tables of scores on the C.M.S. with answers on each aspect of the physical environment

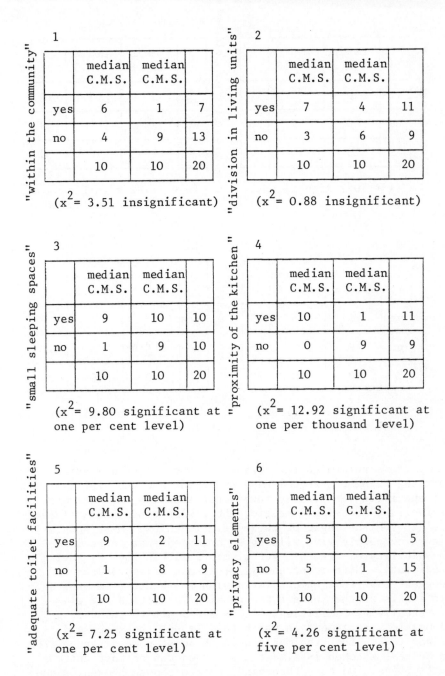

1 — "within the community"

	median C.M.S.	median C.M.S.	
yes	6	1	7
no	4	9	13
	10	10	20

(x^2= 3.51 insignificant)

2 — "division in living units"

	median C.M.S.	median C.M.S.	
yes	7	4	11
no	3	6	9
	10	10	20

(x^2= 0.88 insignificant)

3 — "small sleeping spaces"

	median C.M.S.	median C.M.S.	
yes	9	10	10
no	1	9	10
	10	10	20

(x^2= 9.80 significant at one per cent level)

4 — "proximity of the kitchen"

	median C.M.S.	median C.M.S.	
yes	10	1	11
no	0	9	9
	10	10	20

(x^2= 12.92 significant at one per thousand level)

5 — "adequate toilet facilities"

	median C.M.S.	median C.M.S.	
yes	9	2	11
no	1	8	9
	10	10	20

(x^2= 7.25 significant at one per cent level)

6 — "privacy elements"

	median C.M.S.	median C.M.S.	
yes	5	0	5
no	5	1	15
	10	10	20

(x^2= 4.26 significant at five per cent level)

TABLE 1 (continued)

7

"interior quality"		median C.M.S.	median C.M.S.	
	yes	10	2	12
	no	0	8	8
		10	10	20

(x^2= 10.2 significant at one per cent level)

8

"easy to control env. elements"		median C.M.S.	median C.M.S.	
	yes	10	1	11
	no	0	9	9
		10	10	20

(x^2= 12.92 significant at one per thousand level)

9

"good maintenance"		median C.M.S.	median C.M.S.	
	yes	10	5	15
	no	0	5	5
		10	10	20

(x^2= 4.26 significant at 5 per cent level)

10

"improvements"		median C.M.S.	median C.M.S.	
	yes	5	4	9
	no	5	6	11
		10	10	20

(x^2= 0.02 insignificant)

If we return to the idea of a homelike or domestic setting being the recommended provision and the difficulty of specifying in precise terms what actually characterizes a facility as being domestic, then, with hindsight at least, we can see the logic of these relationships. Most houses in which people live will be so arranged that there is a possibility of control over elements within them by their residents. More importantly, it is not going too far to suggest that that which distinguishes a house from an institution is whether or not the cooking facilities are close to the living facilities. It is difficult to think of a domestic arrangement in which this is not the case, and clear to see that the meals being brought some distance from a central kitchen is almost a sine qua non of institutional activities. On the other hand, people choose houses in many situations vis a vis the community at large. Some prefer to be within the community, others prefer to be on the fringe of it. It is not these overall planning issues which seem to be the critical factors here, but as a number of authors, notably Gunzburg and Gunzburg (1968, 1970) have indicated, it is the details which contribute to the domestication of an institution.

At the very least this material demonstrates that an architectural profile can be drawn which would characterize the physical form of a child oriented or an institution oriented setting. Indeed, a quick estimate could be made of where an institution sat on this dimension by a brief visit using the environment scale, which would predict how child centred the institution would emerge as being on King et al's scale. There are also symbolic qualities apparent from this type of estimate which must have some important role in conceptualization of staff and visitors to these places. For if there are such close correlations between physical form and management practice, experience of the physical form can be used by many people to lead to expectations about the policies and attitudes of the institution. It is not assuming too much of the child residents to believe that they may also be aware of the differences which are so apparent from the study.

SUMMARY AND CONCLUSION

It has been demonstrated, within the limits of the sample studied here, that there is an interlinked set of relationships between how child oriented an institution is, its size and general organization structure and details of its physical environmental arrangements. A lot can be said about institutions for the mentally retarded simply on the basis of whether or not they are a hospital or autonomous units outside of the Health Service system. But even more can be said once knowledge of their size is available.

These results point to the special need to identify organizational structure and management patterns when considering the physical environment. Certainly it is not being suggested that by changing the door knobs or putting the kitchen in a more accessible position that the management practices will also be changed. However, it does suggest that when such provisions are made, certain sorts of practices are more likely to occur. A number of the variables which were found to relate to child management practices were actually under the control of the institution itself, if not in actuality then at least theoretically.

It is therefore possible that the autonomy of the institution, and the smaller scale of those which achieved high scores, encouraged their staff to generate actions or respond to possibilities more readily than their colleagues in less autonomous settings. In these, typically larger, institutions it is likely that staff have to contend with a considerable bureaucracy in order to have any changes carried out. However, it is also possible that the general model, which is behind the Health Service, has readily found its way into mental retardation. The clinical level of cleanliness of the facilities, especially within hospitals, presumably has its impetus from the experiences of hospital wards by the staff, whereas the category (2b) institutions, having a more domestic model to follow were much more concerned with other aspects of running an institution.

This model can have many ramifications. If you are concerned with the effective running of a hospital ward, then having a kitchen nearby can be a distinct disadvantage. If on the other hand you are thinking of your accommodation as providing the basis for a home life for the residents, then it is ludicrous to plan your day around meals that come from some central facility. The theoretical implications, then, for these results are the need to pay more direct attention to the mediating role played by organizational structure in relating physical form to actual day to day practices. Only by dealing with the organization as an entity which can facilitate or interfere with the relationship between physical environment and behaviour can we get a fuller understanding of the way in which an environment can be made more therapeutic.

APPENDIX A

The items of the child management scale
(from King, Raynes and Tizard, 1971)

Rigidity of routine

1. Do the children aged 5 years and over get up at the same
time at weekends as they do during the week?

    0 Different times for all on 2 days
    1 Different for some, or on 1 day only
    2 Same time

2. Do the children aged 5 years and over go to bed at the
same time at weekends as they do during the week?

    0 Different times for all on 2 days
    1 Different for some, or on 1 day only
    2 Same time

3. Do they use the yard or garden at set times?

    0 No, whenever they like
    1 Under various conditions
    2 Yes, set times only

4. Do they use their bedrooms at set times?

    0 No, however they like
    1 Under various conditions
    2 Certain days only

5. Are there set times when visitors can come to the unit?

    0 Any time (except during specified times)
    1 Any day, but set times
    2 Certain days only

6. Which children are routinely toileted at night?

    0 None/some only once
    1 Some more than once
    2 All once or more

'Block treatment'

7. After getting dressed, do the children wait around doing
nothing?

    0 No, they are occupied
    1 Some wait doing nothing
    2 Everybody waits doing nothing

8. Do they wait in line before coming in for breakfast?

    0 None wait
    1 Some wait
    2 All wait

9. Do they wait together as a group before bathing?

    0 None wait, all occupied elsewhere
    1 Some wait, or mixed pattern
    2 All wait

10. Do they wait together as a group after bathing?

    0 None wait, return individually
    1 Some wait, or mixed pattern
    2 All wait

11. How do they return from the toilet?

    0 Individually
    1 In groups, or mixed pattern
    2 All together

12. Do they sit waiting at tables before the meal is served? (tea or evening meal)

    0 Less than 5 minutes (mean day 1 and day 2)
    1 6-10 minutes
    2 More than 10 minutes

13. Do they sit waiting at tables after the meal is finished and before next activity? (tea or evening meal)

    0 Less than 7 minutes (mean day 1 and day 2)
    1 8-14 minutes
    2 15 or more minutes

14. How are the children organized when they go on walks?

    0 Taken a few at a time
    1 All at once, but in separate groups
    2 In 'crocodiles' or similar

Depersonalization

15. What is done with the children's private clothing?

    0 Kept and used by children
    1 Used only on visits, special occasions
    2 Not used or not allowed

16. What is done with the children's private toys?

    0 Kept and used by children
    1 Kept for a time, but become communal
    2 Not used or not allowed

17. How many of the children possess <u>all</u> of the following articles of clothing: shirt or blouse, trousers or skirt, dress or jacket, jumper, topcoat, shoes, dressing gown, slippers?

    0 67% - 100%
    1 34% - 66%
    2 0% - 33%

18. Whereabouts do they keep their daily clothes?

    0 In private provision
    1 In shared provision, supplied weekly
    2 In communal provision, supplied daily

19. How many children have toys or books of their own?

    0 67% - 100%
    1 34% - 66%
    2 0% - 33%

20. Do they have pictures, pin-ups, photos in rooms?

    0 Yes, in all rooms
    1 In some rooms
    2 No

21. How much time do they have for playing?

    0 At least $\frac{1}{2}$ hour each day of observation
    1 At least $\frac{1}{4}$ hour each day of observation
    2 Less than this

22. How are children's birthdays celebrated?

    0 Individual presents or parties
    1 Mixed pattern
    2 Joint parties or no recognition

23. How are tables laid for meals? (tea or evening meal)

    0 Tables laid for all children
    1 Tables laid for some children
    2 Not laid - food and spoon handed out by staff

Note: The term 'private' means clothes or articles provided by parents or relations. For all other items, ownership is not required: it is sufficient for children to have sole, permanent use of the articles, whatever their source, for possession to be established.

Social distance

24. Do the children have any access to the kitchen?

    0   67% - 100%
    1   34% - 66%
    2   0% - 33%

25. Do the children have any access to other areas?

    0   Yes, no restrictions
    1   To some areas
    2   No, doors are kept locked

26. How do staff assist children at toilet times?

    0   One staff member for each child
    1   Mixed pattern
    2   'Conveyor-belt' system

    ('Conveyor-belt' system means that one child passes
    through the hands of two or more members of staff
    during this routine)

27. How do staff assist children at bath times?

    0   One staff member for each child
    1   Mixed pattern
    2   'Conveyor-belt' system

28. Do staff on duty eat with the children?

    0   All staff (at least sometimes)
    1   Some staff, or sit but don't eat
    2   Stand, serve and supervise only

29. Do staff on duty sit and watch TV with children?

    0   Someone usually does
    1   Someone sometimes does
    2   Sporadic supervision only

30. How many children have been on outings with staff in
    the last three months?

    0   67% - 100%
    1   34% - 66%
    2   0% - 33%

REFERENCES

BAKER, A., DAVIES, R. L., SIVADON, P. (1959) Psychiatric
Services and Architecture, World Health Organization,
Public Health Papers No.1, Geneva.

BANK-MIKKELSEN, N. E., et al (1970) The quality of care,
National Society for Mentally Handicapped Children,
London.

BARKER, R. G., GUMP, P. V. (1964) Big School Small School,
Stanford University Press, Stanford, California.

BAYES, K. (1967) The Therapeutic Effect of Environment on
Emotionally Disturbed and Mentally Subnormal Children,
Gresham Press, England.

BETTELHEIM, B. (1974) A Home for the Heart, Thames and
Hudson.

BLAU, P. H. (1956) Bureaucracy in modern society, Random
House, New York.

BLAU, P. H., SCOTT, W. R. (1963) Formal Organizations: A
comparative approach, Routledge and Kegan Paul.

CANTER, D. (1972) "Royal Hospital for Sick Children,
Glasgow: A psychological analysis", The Architects
Journal, 6th September.

CANTER, D. (1975) "Environmental Design and Behaviour", to
be published in the International Encyclopedia of
Neurology, Psychiatry, Psychoanalysis and Psychology.

CLARKE, A. D. B. (1971) Recent advances in the study of
subnormality, National Association for Mental Health,
London.

DENNIS, W., SAYEGH, Y. (1965) "The effect of supplementary experiences upon the behavioural development of infants in institutions", Child Development, 36.

DEPARTMENT OF EDUCATION AND SCIENCE (1972) Designing for the Severely Handicapped, Design Note 10, HMSO, London.

DEPARTMENT OF EDUCATION AND SCIENCE (1974) List of Special Schools for Handicapped Children in England and Wales, HMSO, London.

DEPARTMENT OF HEALTH AND SOCIAL SECURITY (1971) Buildings for Mentally Handicapped People, HMSO, London.

DEPARTMENT OF HEALTH AND SOCIAL SECURITY (1971) Better Services for the Mentally Handicapped, HMSO, London.

DEPARTMENT OF HEALTH AND SOCIAL SECURITY (1971) The Sheffield Development Project, DHSS (mimeo).

DEPARTMENT OF HEALTH AND SOCIAL SECURITY (undated) "A background to design", Hospital Building for the Mentally Handicapped, HMSO, London.

DEPARTMENT OF HEALTH AND SOCIAL SECURITY (undated) "A Hospital Unit for Children", Hospital Building for the Mentally Handicapped, HMSO, London.

DWYBAD, G. (1968) "Changing patterns of residential care for the mentally retarded: A challenge to architecture", First International Congress for the Scientific Study of Mental Deficiency, Montpellier.

ETZIONI, A. (1961) A Comparative Analysis of Complex Organizations, Collier Macmillan.

GOFFMAN, E. (1961) Asylums: Essays on the Social Situation of Mental Patients and other Inmates, Anchor, New York.

GUNZBURG, A. (1968) "Architecture and Mental Subnormality: sensory experiences in the architecture for the mentally subnormal child", Br. J. of Mental Subnormality, 14.

GUNZBURG, H. C., GUNZBURG, A. L. (1970) "Social Education and the Institution: the shaping of a therapeutic 'non institutional environment'", Second Congress of the International Association for the Scientific Study of Mental Deficiency, Warsaw, Poland.

GUNZBURG, H. C., GUNZBURG, A. L. (1973) Mental Handicap and Physical Environment, Bailliere Tindal, London.

GOOD, L., SIEGEL, S., BAY, A. (1965) Therapy by Design, Charles C. Thomas.

HAUN, P. (1950) "Program for a Psychiatric Hospital", Psych. Quart. Suppl., 24.

ITTELSON, W., PROSHANSKY, H., RIVLIN, L. (1970) "The Environmental Psychology of the Psychiatric Ward", in H. Proshansky et al (eds.) Environmental Psychology, Holt, Rinehart and Winston.

ITTELSON et al (1974) An Introduction to Environmental Psychology, Holt, Rinehart and Winston.

KING, R. D., RAYNES, N. W., TIZARD, J. (1971) Patterns of Residential Care: Sociological Studies in Institutions for Handicapped Children, Routledge and Kegan Paul, London.

KIRKBRIDE, T. S. (1880) "On the Construction, Organization and General Arrangements of Hospitals for the Insane", quoted by C. P. Seager, Psychiatry and Architecture: Review of the Literature, The Society of Clinical Psychiatrists, London, 1972.

LINN, L. (1955) "Architecture as Therapy", in A Handbook of Hospital Psychiatry, University Press, New York.

MESMIN, G. (1971) L'enfant, l'architecture et l'espace, Casterman, Paris.

MOOS, R. (1974) Evaluating Treatment Environments, Wiley.

MORRIS, P. (1969) Put Away. A Sociological Study of Institutions of the Mentally Retarded, Routledge and Kegan Paul, London.

NIRJE, B. (1970) "The normalization principle - implications and comments", British Journal of Mental Subnormality, 31.

OSMOND, H. (1970) "Function as the Basis of Psychiatric Ward Design", in W. Proshansky et al (eds.) Environmental Psychology, Holt, Rinehart and Winston.

PARSONS, T. (1960) Structure and Process in Modern Societies, Cass, London.

PAEDIATRIC SOCIETY (1962) The Needs of Mentally Handicapped Children, National Society for Mentally Handicapped Children, London.

RIVLIN, L., WOLFE, M. (1972) "The early history of a psychiatric hospital for children", Environment and Behaviour, March.

SANDHY, Y., HENDRIKS-TANSEY, H. (1976) Environmental Design for Handicapped Children, Saxon House, Farnborough.

TIZARD, B., COOPERMAN, O., JOSEPH, A., TIZARD, J. (1972) "Environmental effects on language development: A study of young children in long stay residential nurseries", Child Development, 43.

ULLMAN, L. P. (1967) Institution and Outcome: A comparative study of psychiatric hospitals, Pergamon Press.

WEEKS, J. (1972) Environment for the Care of Mentally
    Handicapped People, Centre of Environments for the
    Handicapped (mimeo), London.

WING, T. K., BROWN, G. W. (1970) Institutionalism and
    Schizophrenia. A comparative study of three mental
    hospitals, 1960-1968, Cambridge University Press.

WITTMAN, F. D. (1972) "Alcoholism and Architecture: The
    myth of specialized treatment facilities", in Mitchel
    (ed.) EDRA 3, University of California Press.

WOLFE, M. (1975) "Room size, group size and density
    behaviour patterns in a children's psychiatric facility",
    Environment and Behaviour.

'Normal' Environment with a Plus for the Mentally Retarded

H.C. GUNZBURG AND A.L. GUNZBURG

We seem to have passed the distressing stage where, when dealing with the problems of the mentally retarded, we regard them merely as unfortunate biological accidents who are best stored away, 'out of sight, out of mind'. We accept, from the humanitarian point of view, that they should be cared for as well as possible, because they are not able to create a normal existence for themselves. But we also know now that, from the scientific-educational-psychological points of view, they are capable of significant development which will reduce their dependence on other people to a considerable extent. Reducing dependency, or, in more positive terms, increasing independence in the mentally retarded despite their mental disabilities is a formidable task with inherent problems which have never been adequately tackled because few people have appreciated that the development of the mentally retarded to a reasonable level of social functioning requires a comprehensive approach, and even fewer people have had the resources to achieve this approach. Much of the effort towards improving the situation has concentrated on studying the mentally handicapped child's academic difficulties at school and the majority of research work has been devoted to finding a way around the problems of low intelligence and the consequent lack of progress in reading, writing, arithmetic and other school subjects. At work, the mentally retarded adult has recently been found rather less of a problem, provided work demands could be tailored to simple routine; and indeed, it has been shown that with adequate training, many of the more capable mentally retarded people could earn a living, whilst others, less capable, could contribute, often substantially, to their support. The remaining main area proved to be the problems connected with living an 'ordinary' life in the open community, which are far more complex and of a more demanding nature, than those

met either at school or at work. Outside fairly structured
environments, the mentally retarded have found these constantly changing demands very difficult and bewildering.
Some considerable and continuous support seems indeed to be
essential for those mentally retarded persons who can no
longer live in the shelter provided by their immediate
family. In the past this has been given by the institution,
the colony, the hospital, the village; but it has now become
official government policy (Comand No. 4683, "Better Services
for the Mentally Handicapped", H.M.S.O.) that the institutional care of the 'hospital' type should be given only to those
who require 'hospital services' in the true sense of the
word, whilst other mentally handicapped people could be
cared for in non-medical/nursing facilities in the community.

It becomes obvious that the hospital/institution will
have two roles. Firstly, it will continue with a custodial
role for a group of highly dependent mentally handicapped
people, who require hospital/nursing care, and secondly, it
will have to increase its treatment functions in the widest
sense of the term, to make mentally handicapped people fit
better into the life of the normal community. People who
require this type of hospital treatment are those with
severe behaviour disorders and emotional instability who
cannot easily be absorbed into residential facilities without specialist services. The type of treatment required
under those circumstances is partly medical, partly educational, and partly (and probably mainly) experiencing a
structured, reassuring life.

Mentally handicapped people who respond to this approach
will then be discharged into a suitable place in the open
community. To some extent the residential facilities in
the open community - the hostel, the group home - should be
able to reinforce the new life-style acquired in this type
of 'treatment' setting though it will, of necessity, be less
systematic and directive than the work carried out under
optimum conditions.

A therapeutic environment and development

Hospitals/institutions followed by re-introduction to
the community are the environments for many mentally retarded
people today. Yet are they 'Therapeutic Environments'? The
mentally retarded are generally not ill nor out of their
minds, and therapeutic in the sense of restoring a patient
to a state of health previously enjoyed, is not applicable
in their case. If the word refers to contributing to an
acceptable state of well-being, then we get near the common

interpretation of the term. In the place of the shocking
and depressing institutional environments of the past – which
have given the very word institution such a deterring reputation – we find now new, modern, pleasing domestic-like
environments with furniture, curtains and domestic trimmings,
often of a high standard. There is a third meaning to the
word 'therapeutic'. Apart from restoring or contributing
to a state of well-being, it should also develop such a
state. We want to talk about 'therapeutic environment' from
this particular developmental point of view.

AN OPERATIONAL PHILOSOPHY

As was mentioned, the problems of the mentally retarded
nowadays are found in adapting to life and to its perplex-
ities. They have comparatively little mental ability to
handle even simple unfamiliar situations, not to mention
complex ones. Society, in protecting them against the complexities of life, succeeds in depriving them of learning
and practising within a framework of reality.

What we have, in fact, is something of a vicious circle.
The mentally retarded need protection and support because
of their limited mental abilities which, however, could be
stretched much further to their full potential if they did
not have that very protection and support which deprives
them of the opportunity to practise and learn by mistakes.

The over-protection and over-support apparent in our
institutions neatly camouflaged by providing modern comfort,
labour saving devices, domestic staff, canteen facilities,
colour television sets, lounges with larger windows, colour
schemes and soft furnishings – a club atmosphere, relaxing
and pleasant, where people can vegetate in more comfort than
in the past with their cheerless and cold environments
equipped with only the bare essentials.

Is it perhaps possible to make more use of these
physical/environmental elements; to put them to work in the
interest of the mentally retarded so that they are not
merely stored, but also stretched and developed – in the
nicest possible way?

Storage or development

We are putting forward the thesis that a therapeutic
environment for the mentally retarded must provide (a) opportunities for learning within the framework of an educational/

training programme, (b) opportunities for practising skills
within an environment which is 'normal' in the sense that
it reflects some of the ordinary living conditions, and
(c) opportunities for the mentally retarded to develop as
persons who can have likes and dislikes, can choose and
reject and can make meaningful decisions. In short, a
therapeutic environment must provide for the three essential
aspects of development in the mentally retarded:

Socialization (skills of social competence)

Normalization (a 'normal' environment with a plus)

Personalization (application of individuality
within the social context)

The mentally retarded person is, as we all are, a
product of nature and nurture. Research and education/
training specialists have spent many decades of strenuous
effort on alleviating the effects of nature's mistakes in
producing subnormal people. Little attention has been paid
to the effect of nurture, the effects of growing up and
developing within an adverse or beneficial environment.
Nor has much thought been devoted to defining the environment for the mentally retarded person in other than purely
human terms - i.e. the people around him, parents, foster
parents, institution population, staff, teachers etc. The
operational philosophy outlined above under the three headings of Socialization, Normalization and Personalization
requires that the physical factors in the environment - the
design, the architecture - are made an integral part of the
therapeutic environment, because the execution of a developmental programme requires not merely a roof under which
the work is to go on, but a physical structure which supports
the work rather than interferes with it.

Let us explain by giving some practical examples. We
shall refer to the three areas already mentioned, and try
to demonstrate how the inclusion of certain features in the
design will help to create the helpful framework of a therapeutic environment. It will obviously also depend on the
people working with the mentally retarded to make full use
of the opportunities created. It cannot be emphasized too
often that the developmental process of stretching the
mentally retarded's abilities to the full, must be done
systematically by the people working there, and that the
physical environment by itself will have little influence
in development unless it is properly interpreted and used.

Much attention has been focused on the mentally retarded person's deficiencies in motivation and communication. No doubt these deficiencies are very real ones and are basic to the condition of mental retardation. These inherent deficiencies in mental retardation lead to a handicap, just as a physical deficiency, such as blindness and the loss of a limb result in a handicap compared with people who can see and have the use of all their limbs. If nothing is done to make such a person function better despite the defect, the handicap may become so dominant that the person's whole life style deteriorates. On the other hand, a successful remediation of the handicap may give such a person a nearly normal life.

We must really learn to think of the mentally retarded in the same way. There is the defect - nothing much can be done about it - but the handicap, resulting from the defect, can be reduced or increased by adequate or inadequate measures. One of these measures is the physical environment. Is the environment therapeutic if it is adjusted to the mentally retarded's handicap to make it easier for him, or is it therapeutic if it is designed to make demands on him, despite his handicap?

Now, let us look at some of the physical features which interfere with the creation of a therapeutic environment.

SOCIALIZATION

This aspect refers particularly to skills of social competence such as self-help, communication, socialization and occupation skills, which must be systematically taught and practised to achieve a reasonable degree of social independence.

It is not widely enough appreciated by administrators, educationists and designers that social learning must be done in context and not be limited to the carefully super-vised unnatural setting of domestic science centres, social education rooms or even education flats etc. Whilst these facilities are needed to initiate the learning process, because they are designed as a learning environment with a supervising teaching staff, the mentally retarded require consolidation through a learning environment which is 'there' after formal instruction has stopped. Efforts by educationists, psychologists, trainers, are a complete waste of time if there is no possibility for the mentally retarded to transfer the skills acquired in one setting to another

setting, because the regulations do not permit it, the staff
do not encourage it or the building design does not provide
the opportunities.

If it has been thought desirable and appropriate that
the mentally handicapped person should learn to prepare a
snack for himself, to put the kettle on and make tea, to
lay the table and this is formally taught in one setting,
then his home life, whether it is hostel or hospital ward,
must provide the facilities to apply what he has learnt.
He must have access to a small kitchen, where he must be
permitted to deal with hot and cold water taps, he must be
given space for his food store, he must be expected to lay
the table and serve himself. These seem to be very obvious
and perhaps, at first glance, not very controversial points -
yet community hostels are built with big hygienic kitchens,
accessible to residents only under supervision, safety regulations in hospitals forbid the introduction of hot water
taps, and food is being served by domestic and nursing
personnel because it is easier and less time consuming.
Indeed, a good many potentially very useful social learning
situations in a domestic setting are discarded by the designer from the outset because there are other more time-saving
and economical solutions for dealing efficiently with groups
of people. This seems to us to negate the requirements of
a therapeutic environment for the individual mentally retarded person in favour of an impersonal administrative arrangement, which provides only the acceptable standards of storing
people where they can feed, sleep and wash, when they are
not required elsewhere for some form of education, treatment
and training.

An integrated therapeutic environment for the mentally
handicapped must be conceived not only as giving further
opportunities for practising social skills painfully and
slowly acquired and formally taught, but must also, as much
as possible, elicit responses by avoiding making life so
simple that it furthers a vegetating existence. A wide corridor makes it easy to go from A to B without noticing whom
one passes - a narrower one forces attention on to the other
person and perhaps also application of the skills of 'social
graces' by saying "excuse me" and "sorry".

The design of public areas to provide plenty of space
for a group of people will sometimes look good from an
aesthetic point of view and makes it easy for the domestic
worker to get round it with a huge industrial vacuum cleaner
and polisher. But this architectural solution results not
only in a loss of domestic atmosphere (substituting it by a
permanent clubroom life) but deprives the residents of the
experience and daily routine of cleaning up their own terri-
tories.

We would argue that the environment must provide as
many learning opportunities as possible, which will encourage
a development of those aspects of poor motivation and poor
communication which still represent great problems of adjustment. Television viewing is made comfortable because there
are twenty-five chairs pertinently placed by the interior
designers for the twenty-five residents. The same television
programme could, however, be used for motivating people to
fetch chairs from elsewhere in order to sit comfortably -
a perfectly normal routine, requiring moreover the acquisition of the additional domestic habit of returning the
chairs after the event and restoring the room to its original
state.

So far as communication is concerned, this is not only
by words and sight, but by smell, taste and feeling. How
many of those additional channels of communication are we
neglecting by eliminating in our design solution the possibilities of domestic aromas when the central kitchen provides everything ready cooked, and when perfumed soaps,
toilet water, after shave etc. are ruled out on principle
by the administrator? Or, when we fail to provide all those
different tasty sauces and other extras for the dining table?
Or when the whole building uses the same serviceable floor
covering, paint and upholstery? These are small details
which the architect, administrator, finance officer, do not
regard as important in their attempt to provide quickly and
economically a decent roof and shelter. Yet, these are the
small, all-important details which make up the life of
persons whose interests centre around their immediate surroundings - often not more than a room, a building. If the
designer were to introduce right from the beginning those
features which require different treatment in texture, which
give different vistas and which provide interest and home-
liness by being related to the mentally retarded person's
world, then this will become, in the hands of the right
people, a therapeutic environment which stretches and demands
a response, rather then acquiesces to the handicap.

At this point we would like to introduce the concept of
'normalization' as applied to the physical environment.

NORMALIZATION

We are talking primarily of the creation of a 'normal
physical environment' which will further the development of
social and personal skills.

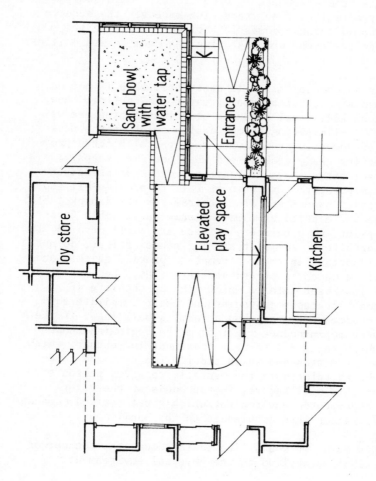

Figure 1: Play space environment for very young children in domestic setting

Normalization is, seen in our terms, a selective procedure which emphasizes those features of normal life which
will help the mentally retarded person to develop his potential.

There is nowadays such an overflow of 'institutional'
features into normal life patterns (such as ready-packed,
plated meals) that it is easy to justify the introduction
of these impersonal, dehumanised features into hostel and
hospital life in the name of 'normality'. Yet, these features (e.g. throw away plastic cutlery and paper plates) are
not part of the domestic atmosphere nor are they capable of
development in the sense of adding the personal refinements
expressing likes and dislikes. It will be essential to
select in planning and management those features which help
in developing the mentally retarded, rather than those which
provide a convenient solution for dealing with his deficiencies. Such a selection is of necessity an arbitrary process
and must be governed by what we know of the mentally retarded
person's abilities. Since, for example, we wish to increase
his communication skills, we feel that realistic pictures
which have some immediate meaning to him, will be more helpful than any abstract paintings, murals, etc. His appreciation of colour and patterns will often be different from
that of the senior staff and wallpapers and colour schemes
should be chosen for his enjoyment rather than be selected
by the nursing officers and architects to their personal
taste.

Normalization of this type requires also from the
designer a little more imagination in providing such important living spaces as one's bedroom. Instead of taking the
easy way of stringing out a row of identical rooms on either
side of a corridor, and leaving it to the interior designer
to differentiate them by the use of green and pink colour
schemes, variety must be brought into the design right from
the beginning. There must be rooms of different appearances
to choose from - some which are larger and take two beds,
others are one bedded rooms, have windows in different positions, have little alcoves etc. and have, in short, different atmospheres which will help to make one bedroom look
quite different from the bedroom next door.

Why should a dining room be always so functional and
efficient that it can compete with the factory canteen and
with any modern high speed food dispensing organization?
Normal, yes, but therapeutic in the sense of developing a
person, no! This type of environment is not favoured in a
home and it is not permitted in the pub or in those dining

places where one is prepared to pay something extra for domestic warm comfort. Each of these dining out places proves every evening that one can feel comfortable in a crowded room, that one can get stimulated by vision and taste and that food can be served to a considerable number of people even if it means having to squeeze through closely placed chairs – so why make the dining space for the mentally retarded only convenient for staff and unstimulating for the residents?

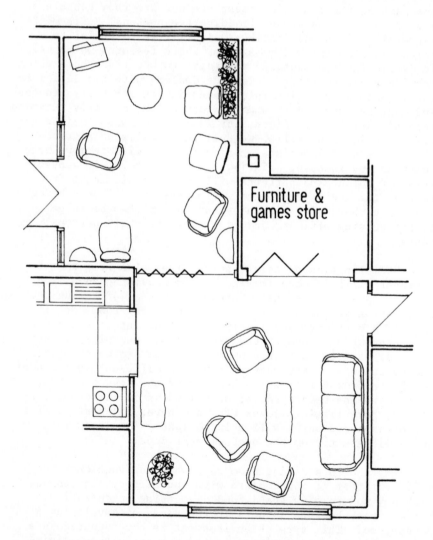

Figure 2: Living space for teenage and grown up people in domestic setting

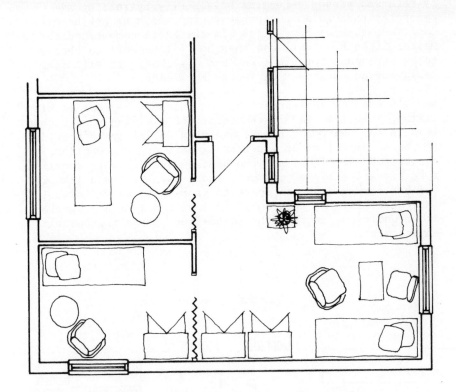

Figure 3:   Bedroom for all ages in domestic setting

PERSONALIZATION

And this leads quite naturally to the aspect of person-alization, which can only result from the successful combin-ation of socialization and normalisation. Only when the training in social skills has achieved a reasonable level of competence so that the mentally retarded person is not bogged down with his own technical inefficiency; only when he has adjusted to living in a normal environment which provides him daily with opportunities for learning and prac-tising (hence the 'normal environment with a plus') will he have acquired the necessary fundamental habits and knowledge to develop as a person.

Personalization refers, therefore, to that aspect which cannot be taught directly, but which shows quite clearly once a person is neither hemmed in by his own ignorance and incompetence nor has to take evasive action by withdrawal,

flight or aggression. Once we have achieved giving a mentally retarded person a feeling of security by guiding him
carefully through an environment with which he has become
familiar, then we have given him the basic competence to
master it on his level and then he will be able to choose,
to have reasons for his likes and dislikes, and will make
decisions on the basis of secure knowledge.

In such an environment he can choose a bedroom to his
liking, select a seat in the corner of a dining room rather
than in the centre, can make use of a social space provided
by the architect at an interesting part of the corridor,
can switch the lights and the heat on and off when required,
make himself a cup of tea or a snack when he feels like it
and has enough cupboard space to store his individual belongings near him. In such conditions he can live and develop.
Such conditions provide the foundations for a therapeutic
environment.

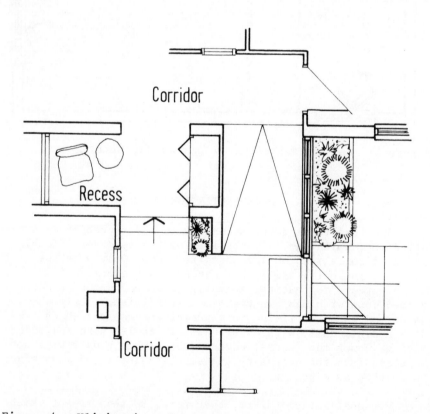

Figure 4: Ulitization of corridor space as "fun area" for
older children in domestic setting

CONCLUDING REMARKS

Some of the features discussed in this paper were published some time ago in a paper under the title "39 steps leading towards normalized living practices in Living Units for the Mentally Handicapped". It provided a checklist of thirty-nine features which we regarded as minimal to start the ball rolling. In that list, some of the decisions to be made are not in the hands of the designers - e.g. whether the bathroom in a training area should have mixing valve or hot and cold taps, whether toilets in such areas should offer adequate normal privacy. But other small details can be incorporated into the design right at the beginning to show, so to speak, the correct way to the future users, both staff and residents, e.g. a mirror in the bedroom and near the front door, shelves, hooks in the bathroom, toilets, bedroom, variety of light fittings, different types of chairs and a greater variety of furniture. The problem in many ways is simply that of realizing that the physical environment can be a therapeutic tool if the treatment philosophy accepts that treatment in 'learning to live skills' requires the right type of environment. As long as the architect and designer look at their task mainly as one of providing the best possible shell for housing so and so many people for so and so many activities, there will be no therapeutic environment in the sense of a developing environment.

In the approach we have outlined there is no mystique, no wonderful therapy which will cure the mentally retarded. But we have no doubt that a large number of the mentally retarded are so under-functioning at present that we shall see them as quite different persons, and more capable persons, once we have given them a chance to develop properly. Putting up a therapeutic environment for the mentally retarded provides a better type of framework for work, education and training and the staff will have to learn to take advantage of what is carefully incorporated in the design.

It is probably easier to attract people's attention by extolling the therapeutic advantages of special shapes, sizes and colours which, by the very fact that something special is introduced, have some extra persuasiveness. We feel, however, there is no need to add 'foreign' and 'alien' aspects to the world surrounding the mentally handicapped and that the emphasis must be on the selection of helpful ordinary 'normal' elements which will make the mentally handicapped feel 'at home'. A therapeutic environment is not achieved simply by leaving out all those aspects which are obviously 'ab-normal', e.g. large dayrooms, dormitories.

Creating a therapeutic environment for the mentally handicapped requires a sensitive appraisal of the relevance and significance of normal elements - and this task of selection needs an understanding for the developmental issues applicable to the whole range of mental handicap, as well as imagination and sympathy.

READINGS ON ENVIRONMENT AND MENTAL HANDICAP

by

H. C. Gunzburg and A. L. Gunzburg

The "Living Unit" - A New Design for the Long Stay Patient
(1961) in J. Ment. Subn., 7.13, pp.73-79.

Architecture for Social Rehabilitation (1967) in J. Ment.
Subn., Vol.13, pp.84-87.

Sensory Experiences in the Architecture for the Mentally
Subnormal Child (1968) in J. Ment. Subn., Vol.14,
pp.57-58.

The Nurse and Institutional Design in Mental Subnormality
Hospitals (1970) in Nursing Times, 10, pp.121-124.

Practice in Living (1970) in British Hospital Journal and
Social Service Review, November, pp.2274-2276.

Subnormality - in Integrated Service (1971) in Nursing
Mirror, March, pp.34-38.

Social Education and the Institution: The Shaping of a
Therapeutic "Non-Institutional" Environment (1971) in
Proceedings of 2nd Congress of IASSMD Warsaw, Polish
Medical Publishers, pp.175-180.

Social Development and Architectural Planning in Hospital
and Community (1971) in Proceedings of 2nd Congress of
IASSMD Warsaw, Polish Medical Publishers, pp.610-611.

From Ward to Living Unit. A pilot scheme in reshaping the
mental subnormality hospital (1971) in Brit. J. M. Subn.,
17.32, pp.54-65.

39 Steps Leading Towards Normalized Living Practices in Living Units for the Mentally Handicapped (1973) in Brit. J. Ment. Subn., Vol.19, No.37, pp.91-99.

Mental Handicap and Physical Environment (1973) Bailliere Tindall, London.

The effect of a new improved physical environment on the implementation of a normalizing programme (1973) Unpublished report, Birmingham Subnormality Division.

The Physical Environment as a Supportive Factor in Rehabilitation (1974) in Experiments in the Rehabilitation of the Mentally Handicapped (ed. H. C. Gunzburg), Butterworths, London.

The Hospital Living Unit - Comfortable Storage or Intensive Treatment Area? (1974) in Apex, Vol.2, No.1, pp.1-7.

The Search for a Home Environment (1974) in Brit. J. Ment. Subn., XX, 38, pp.28-42.

Units for the Mentally Handicapped (1974) Stratford Upon Avon, IDC.

Children's Units in Hospitals for the Mentally Handicapped - Some findings relating to Architectural Briefing (1976) in Brit. J. Ment. Subn., Vol.22, 42, pp.47-51.

The Design of a Therapeutic Children's Residential Unit (1976) in REAP, Vol.2, p.3.

A Therapeutic Environment for Forensic Patients

JONATHAN D. SIME AND DAVID A. SIME

INTRODUCTION

The report of the Butler Committee (1974) highlighted the need, when dealing with forensic psychiatric patients, to reconcile public safety with the desire for the most appropriate treatment for individual offenders. They proposed that a forensic unit be something between a hospital and a prison, in that a treatment concept is vital as a primary aim but the public also have to be protected; hence adequate surveillance remains an important issue.

This chapter considers one unit which has attempted to provide a facility such as that proposed by the Butler Committee. It is hoped that by presenting the details of the operation of such a unit that the strengths and weaknesses of the concept of the forensic unit can be evaluated.

The unit studied was established in a mentally handicapped hospital in 1968 with the following aims, as delineated by the consultant psychiatrist originally responsible for the development of the unit (the co-author of this paper).

1. To create a therapeutic environment with a mutual support system between staff and patients.

2. To run the unit on multi-disciplinary lines and to encourage outside professionals and therapists to work in the unit.

3. To test out the effects of such management in an open unlocked modern unit.

4.   To develop an appropriate environment and milieu towards the rehabilitation of the abnormal offender.

5.   To create an ethos in which the individual himself is very much involved in the working out of his own problems under guidance towards a sensible future.

6.   To exclude low intelligence per se as an indicator for admission.

7.   To test out the degree to which a variety of cases can be managed in an open unit (including offenders who have committed serious offences e.g. arsonists, sexual and violent offenders etc.).

It should be noted that the term 'patient' has been used to refer to the individual in the unit. This reflects its hospital and treatment orientation, as opposed to a custodial and penal one, although practically every inmate was originally admitted to the unit through the courts.

A further primary aim of the unit was to test out the management of a range of difficult behaviour disorders in a new building, using a regime based on encouraging patients to participate in their own management (peer group management). Individual counselling, group therapy techniques and regular work are considered to be important. Other aspects of the management process include techniques towards raising self-esteem.

The therapeutic management concepts are based partly on the experience of one of the consultants at Grendon Psychiatric Prison and elsewhere, and partly in relation to the management requirements of an open unit. Another consultant, who joined the unit later, also had extensive forensic psychiatric experience in prisons. To some degree its therapeutic aims have been additionally influenced by the building setting itself. This will be clarified in the following sections.

HISTORY OF THE UNIT

Details of the origins of the unit, its current use and user reactions to it were collected through informal interviews with the architect, staff and patients as well as from existing records and reports (Sime and Easby, 1973, Frankenburg and Millham, 1976). 23 interviews were carried out with patients and 24 with staff (cf. Sime, 1975 for details). The interviews supplemented data provided by the observational studies described later.

The original ward for behaviour disturbance

The Prentice Unit in Langdon Hospital, Devon, evolved originally out of another ward, Dart Ward. Dart Ward, which stands on the same campus, had been a locked ward with a high proportion of delinquent subnormal patients. Built in the 1930's, its design was based on the standard, two-storey institutional villa pattern of the time. It is one of a row of similar villas and is characterised by its large regimented dormitory area, ward dayroom and a general absence of single room facilities.

The staff of this originally locked ward had found it more and more difficult in later years to cope with patients and their damage to the interior decor, furniture and the windows. The atmosphere of the ward may have been aggravated by over-crowding. At about that time it was considered that changes were needed because of the somewhat unsatisfactory social and physical conditions in the ward, and also because of problems of morale in its staff and patients. Coincidentally, a newly built ward had become available, the Prentice Ward. The Prentice Ward had originally been designed for mentally handicapped patients of fairly limited intelligence. Before its commission, however, it had been decided to use it to house patients from a ward in another hospital which was to be demolished. In view of the difficulties on Dart Ward it was decided to decant the more difficult and brighter patients from Dart 'Villa', together with other court cases from the rest of the hospital group. The (60 bedded) Prentice Unit was thus a forensic unit from the beginning.

The new building

In a recent interview with the architect he explained that because the new building, completed in 1968, was originally designed to cater for low grade subnormal patients, it was greatly influenced by guidance subsequently available in Building Note 32, published by the Ministry of Health (1964). The building was thus not primarily designed by the architect for the type of forensic patient that now uses it. Its physical design with its large ground floor layout and modern, spacious appearance is a clear contrast to the original Dart Ward building, and indeed also to a prison

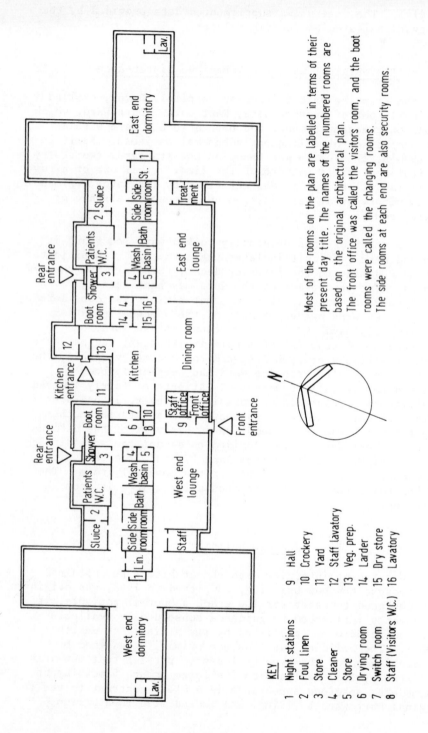

Most of the rooms on the plan are labelled in terms of their present day title. The names of the numbered rooms are based on the original architectural plan.

The front office was called the visitors room, and the boot rooms were called the changing rooms.

The side rooms at each end are also security rooms.

KEY

1 Night stations
2 Foul linen
3 Store
4 Cleaner
5 Store
6 Drying room
7 Switch room
8 Staff (Visitors W.C.)
9 Hall
10 Crockery
11 Yard
12 Staff lavatory
13 Veg. prep.
14 Larder
15 Dry store
16 Lavatory

Figure 1: The Prentice Unit: ground floor plan

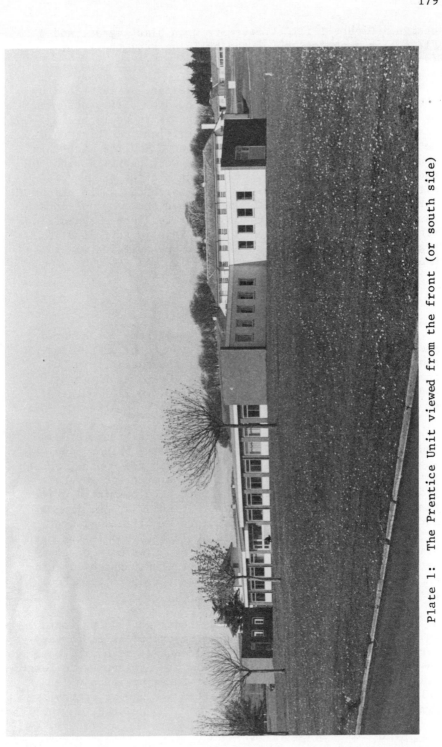

Plate 1: The Prentice Unit viewed from the front (or south side)

design. Figure 1 illustrates its open plan layout, and Plate 1 is a photograph of the building from the front (south side).

The overriding concept of the design, as described by the architect, was that 'patients could be easily observed by staff'. It was considered that patients would be in need of a lot of attention and supervision and this would be facilitated by the open plan layout. In line with this emphasis, 'Nightingale Ward' layouts were provided with the beds set out in rows. In this design a night station is situated in a central position from which the whole of the dormitory can be seen. It appears that the original concept was for two 30-bed units to be integrated into a symmetrical plan with a dormitory at each end. This is reflected in Figure 1. The architect stated that the building was to be made as 'non-institutional as possible'.

The patients

By January 1973 it is recorded that some two hundred and fifty-eight patients had been through the unit (Sime and Easby, 1973). Only sixty-one of the patients in the sample up to 1973 had an IQ of below 70 and at the other end of the scale fifteen had an IQ of above 110. Generally, as Frankenberg and Millham (1976) indicate in a re-analysis of existing records for this period up to 1973, Prentice tends to have had more young patients and patients of a lower average IQ than would be found in the prison population. The average length of stay up to 1973 was ten months, though in some cases patients have been in the unit for several years. Patients admitted to the unit have committed crimes ranging from sex offences, theft, violence, arson, drug and motor offences. There have been more sexual and violent offenders in its population than would be found in the open prisons (Frankenberg and Millham 1976). Yet more of these patients had pursued a 'medical career' through child guidance and mental hospitals rather than the approved school system.

At the time of the 1975 study there were 46 patients in the unit. 27 of these might be described as short-stay (arbitrarily defined in the present context as having been in the unit for less than one year). 19 patients were long-stay (more than one year). Most of these patients were below the age of 30 and had committed a range of crimes similar to those reflected in the earlier records.

Selection procedures

During the nine years of the unit's existence, every case has been pre-seen by one or other of the two consultants associated with the unit. Most of these admissions have related to a court appearance where prison would have been the alternative disposal. Selection on the basis of a genuine wish on the part of the individual for help is attempted but this is to an extent clouded by the prison alternative.

In the 1973 study, out of 258 cases, 62 were Section 60 admissions, 14 were Section 65 admissions (Mental Health Act, 1959), 121 were admitted under a probation order with a condition of residence, and 47 were informal admissions. In practice a probation order has been increasingly found to be the better form of admission. There is more thorough and longer after-care through the probation service. There is a voluntary element implicit in the original order, but the patient can be returned to court again if he is found to be beyond control.

The careful selection of staff has been considered to be of fundamental importance to the successful running of the unit. Prentice has been particularly fortunate in this respect, in the consultant's opinion, with excellent nursing leadership and high quality staff. Despite this, as will be seen later, institution communication problems have been evident from time to time.

PEOPLE AND SETTING

In trying to characterise the fit between the people and their physical setting, three broad indices are worthy of consideration: damage, absconding, and change of use.

a) Damage to old and new buildings

Despite the fact that much of the information provided here on the development of the unit is retrospective in nature, the interview material does suggest that damage done to the old Dart Ward was a reaction in part against the over-crowded and restrictive conditions. The absence of over-crowding in the Prentice Unit, together with changes in the social organisation, have no doubt contributed to the reduction in damage and the better management of the patients. Changes in the social organisation include improved staff-patient relations, different rules from the old ward and a different balance in the types of patients admitted. At the same time the greater vigilance, ease of observation and open door policy (freedom of access to the hospital grounds) afforded by the newer building's design, contributed to the unit's development. Patients appear to have had greater pride in the new building and peer group influence towards increased tidiness was actively encouraged from the start.

b) Absconding and the open plan

The belief in the importance of the open plan building design to the therapeutic aims of the unit was reflected in interview statements by both staff and patients. Thus one member of staff had this to say: "The open plan is very important. In a secure unit people are utterly demoralised. You can't socialise a man by locking him up". A similar sentiment was expressed by a patient: "The open plan helps in a way. It gives a bloke freedom and peace of mind. Locked up in a cell you always start to bear a grudge." However, this openness does provide greater possibilities for absconding. Nonetheless, the figures which are available reveal that it has been generally possible to manage often very difficult patients in it. Records for a sample of 161 of the patients admitted to the unit between July 1968 and October 1972 reveal that 51% did not abscond, 31% absconded either once or twice and the remainder three or more times (Frankenberg and Millham, 1976). In this context absconding means any unauthorised absence from the hospital campus, including late return from parole, leave etc. In this sense, an 'environmental/learning theory' view of absconding may be more appropriate than an 'internal causality' theory. Clarke and Martin (1975) have suggested this in their research of approved schools (also open plan). Variations in absconding behaviour were found to be more a function of the nature of the school regime than of the characteristics of residents. The present research suggests that the physical setting contributes to the factors which encourage absconding, for example the quality and degree of interaction with members of staff, and visits from outside, as well as the opportunities for escape.

During the last two years particular efforts have been made to tackle the problem of absconding, both by selecting out the serious potential absconder in relation to previous patterns of behaviour and also by tightening up the rules over absconding in general. This approach appears to have made a definite impact on the problem, although figures are not yet available.

c) Changes to the building

A consideration of the functional changes made within, or to, the building is another way of considering the relation between the occupants and their environment. It might be thought that the effective development of the unit would have depended on a number of modifications being made to the facility. There have been few functional changes to the building itself since the unit opened. Those which have occurred include the slight modification of two of the side rooms and a change in function of the front office from a visitor's room to one which the unit nursing officer and consultants occupy from time to time. There have been unsuccessful attempts to run the unit as two sub-wards in line with the symmetrical layout of the building. The two night stations were used as sub unit staff offices with the central staff office providing a link between the two sides. Patients were kept in their separate halves. This was abandoned, however, due to organisational and communication problems between the two halves. Recently, an unsuccessful attempt was made to change the usage of the treatment room into an additional consulting room. Latterly, the size of the unit has been considered to be a critical factor and the numbers have been gradually reduced from 60 to 45. There was a consensus belief that this led to better patient management.

The general lack of physical or functional changes to the building appears to indicate a good fit between the people and the setting. However, deficiencies of the building may be masked since it is apparent that people can adapt to aspects of a physical setting which may not be optimal. In addition, administrative constraints limit the number of changes which are possible. The observational data is therefore necessary to further explore this theme. Indications of the need for this other data come from another study carried out at almost the same time as the present one (Hudson, 1976). She emphasized the problems in communication and a certain lack of cohesion within different groups of staff and between some staff and the patients. This was despite the emphasis which is placed on the relationships between the staff and patients towards changing attitudes and behaviour. Listing Clark's three criteria for a therapeutic milieu, freedom, activity and responsibility (Clark, 1974), she referred to the substantial freedom allowed, but noted a lack of organised activity and limitations in responsibility afforded to patients.

The remainder of this chapter, then, will be concerned with considering the level at which the unit actually

functions by establishing the patterns of activity which
characterise it. In broad terms we shall consider whether
this level of functioning is optimal or appropriate in terms
of the therapeutic aims and the way in which the physical
environment is used.

THE OBSERVATIONS OF PEOPLE AND ACTIVITIES

The approach adopted to the study of activities in the
unit is comparable with that used in previous 'behavioural
mapping' studies (Ittelson et al, 1970 a). The emphasis in
this work has been on establishing the consistent patterns
in the utilisation of different areas of the physical settings of psychiatric facilities.

As the first stage of the 'mapping' study, certain
characteristic descriptive items need to be selected which
would summarise the basic patterns of activity throughout
the unit. While these had to be representative, they were
limited in number so as to make it practicable for the
researcher to handle them when the observations were actually
being carried out.

Categories of activity were first drawn up by adapting
the list used in a previous behavioural mapping study of
three psychiatric hospitals (Ittelson et al, 1970 a, p.661).
This list was modified on the basis of a pilot observation
study and interviews. Many of the items were redefined
(Table 1). The present approach differs from the descriptive
selection procedure used by Ittelson et al, where items are
condensed from observers' descriptive records of the setting.
One of the functions of the interviews was to establish the
kinds of activities which the occupants felt they themselves
habitually indulged in. The advantage of this approach was
in making it less likely that initial interpretations of the
range of activities by an observer might bias the item selection procedure.

The method of observation was one of 'time sampling'
every 20 minutes throughout the building complex. Using a
sequential procedure, the observer moved through the whole
building over a strictly controlled 20 minute period, so
that observations were made at regular intervals in each of
eight designated areas. As only one observer was involved
observations could not be made simultaneously in the different areas. The observer used the categories of behaviour
to mark down on a transparent sheet, placed over various
section maps of the unit, the relative positions and activities of the occupants.

Table 1:
Categories of behaviour used in the observational study

SYMBOL	CATEGORY	DESCRIPTION OF BEHAVIOUR: EXAMPLES
○	TALK	Talk or listening. Interaction between individuals.
⊖	GAMES	Cards, scrabble, darts or table tennis.
▲	WATCHING	Watching an activity, people looking outside.
△ (with horizontal line)	READING	Reading or writing (a book, paper, letter, report).
■	PERSONAL	Personal behaviour. Washing hands, having a bath, cleaning clothes, ironing, dressing/undressing.
●	SLEEP/ LYING AWAKE	Sleeping or lying awake on an arm-chair or bed.
◨	SITTING/ STANDING PASSIVE	Inactive or passive behaviour, e.g. sitting/standing alone.
◐	TELEVISION	Watching television.
⊕	MUSIC	Listening to the radio, gramophone, playing the guitar.
□	EATING	Eating or drinking. Patients eating meal, staff drinking coffee.
△	TRAFFIC	Walking through a room or area, standing in a queue.
⊞	SITTING/ STANDING ACTIVE	Making a model, looking for something, taking out objects from a cupboard.
⊠	HOSPITAL ROUTINE	Organisational duties. Staff dispensing drugs, unlocking doors, patient making bed, cleaning.

A total of 125 observation periods (41 hours, 40 minutes) was covered over a period of 10 days from a Thursday
to the following Sunday week. It was considered that a
total coverage of the patients' 'waking hours' from 7 a.m.
to 11 p.m. would be most appropriate to the aims of the
study. This might most accurately represent the way in
which the unit functions. It differs from a coverage of
the 'peak hours' which has characterised other behavioural
mapping studies (Ittelson et al, 1970, a, b, Rivlin and
Wolfe, 1972). Results of the mapping were superimposed on
plans of the building layout so that the people and activities could be clearly related to the architectural plan of
the building. The maps therefore represent the activity
patterns and characteristic occupant locations at different
times of the day and week and over the total period.

If an activity was noted in a location on more than 1
out of 6 of the total number of observations for that period,
then it is included on the final activity 'map' or plan. A
limitation of the present approach is that information
might be lost about changes within any one area of the
building, or activities which take a short length of time.
Material from the interviews made it possible to draw out
other patterns of activity which might otherwise have been
lost.

If we now turn to the behavioural maps for the total
period of observations (Figures 2 and 3), a number of features which characterise the occupants' use of the building
can be summarised. (Details of the daily and weekend activities are available in Sime, 1975.)

Staff and patient areas

Although the term 'open plan' is applied to the unit
by both the staff and patients, the different degree to
which people occupy particular areas reflects a clear distinction between staff and patient areas. Since an aim of
the unit is to encourage mutual support and interaction
between patients and staff, the division between these areas
would appear to be therapeutically counter-productive.

Figure 2 shows that members of staff tend to spend much
of their time in the staff office and to some extent in the
front office. As the interviews with staff suggested, much
of their activity in other areas involves passing through
the building rather than remaining in a single spot. This
movement of the staff is under-represented in the present

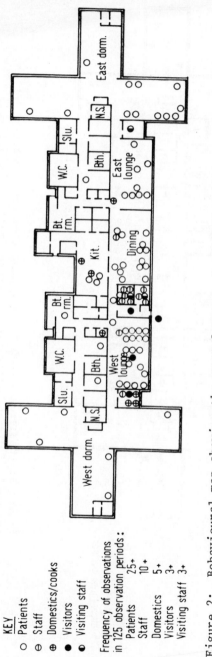
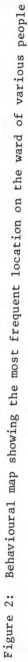

KEY

○ Patients
⊖ Staff
⊕ Domestics/cooks
● Visitors
◉ Visiting staff

Frequency of observations
in 125 observation periods:

Patients   25+
Staff   10+
Domestics   5+
Visitors   3+
Visiting staff   3+

West dorm. N.S. Slu. W.C. Bt. rm. Kit. Bt. rm. W.C. Slu. East dorm.

West lounge Bth. Dining East lounge Bth. N.S.

Figure 2:   Behavioural map showing the most frequent location on the ward of various people

188

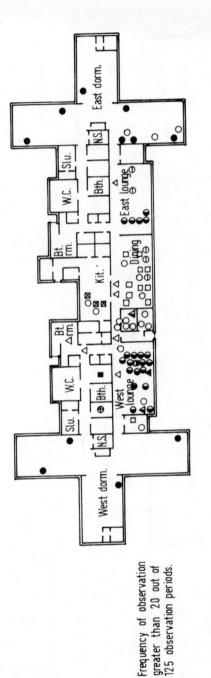

Frequency of observation
greater than 20 out of
125 observation periods.

Figure 3: Behavioural map showing most frequent location
on the ward of various activities for total period (see Table 1)

map. It might be noted that although the staff were some-times seen in the focal areas of the unit, they were rarely seen in the dormitories, that part of the unit which is furthest from the front office.

The fact that the unit does have a focal area which has as its centre the staff office is a positive factor. The staff office tends to get over-crowded, however. The staff complained in interviews that individual private counselling of patients was difficult there and throughout the building generally. It was also clear that although a number of patients do approach the staff in this room and there are advantages in that members of staff can be found there, there are still patients who are reluctant to intrude into or approach this area of staff territory.

Figure 2 also illustrates that visitors tend to collect at the entrance to the building. One of the main recommend-ations in the interviews was that a visitors' room should be provided for patients. The visiting staff (probation officers, consultants, etc.) are even more likely to remain in the staff rooms than any of the other groups. The visiting staff rarely use the staff room (St) however, which is a meeting point for the domestics but not the cooks, who remain in the kitchen. The kitchen tends to be a separate part of the unit altogether. The only patients using it are those whose job it is to work there. It is possible that for these patients this area is similar to the 'free places' Goffman describes (Goffman, 1961).

In fact the results generally support the work of Goffman in relation to institutional settings, which implies that staff/patient role differences are reflected in both the psychological and physical barriers to social discourse (Goffman, 1961). Lecompte (1972), too, has found differences in hospital settings in the amount to which doctors, nurses and therapists filled the 'front-stage' (where patients are) or 'back-stage' (from which patients are excluded). The variable use of staff rooms by different staff members may also reflect other organisational barriers to communication between the different staff groups themselves. Hudson referred in her study of the unit (Hudson, 1976) to the gaps in communication between different nursing shifts. The present interviews indicated that the main source of conten-tion between visiting and nursing staff was in who should have primary access to certain staff rooms. During the study, competition for rooms was normally avoided by offer-ing the treatment room to visiting staff, and arranging for them to visit the unit at different times.

Predominant activities

The predominance of activities such as television watching in the lounges, eating in the dining room and sleeping or lying awake in the dormitories, is a reflection of certain 'constraints' on the patients' activities. These constraints on activity in certain areas are 'psychological' in that patients and staff may feel inhibited from performing certain activities in other people's presence, or remaining for long in a given area. In some cases it has become acceptable for certain activities to take place only at certain times of day. Functional constraints such as the layout of the furniture, or physical barriers such as the locking of the treatment room all reflect aspects of organisational control over the activities.

The colour television has an important effect on behaviour. Even when it is not on, patients can be seen sitting in rows and it is unusual for them to rearrange this furniture. The effect of television in so far as the unit is concerned is to make it a 'more manageable' one. On the other hand, it inhibits other behaviour and may reduce the 'recipient' to a passive role, rather than encourage the active self-reliant one which the unit appears to want to foster. The division between the kitchen and dining room also reduces the degree to which patients can learn to be self-sufficient or responsible.

Degree of privacy

The balance between public and more private areas has been noted in other studies of therapeutic environments, such as Rivlin and Wolfe's behavioural mapping study of a children's hospital (Rivlin and Wolfe, 1972). It is a balance which appears to characterise certain environmental settings and social organisations. It could have been that its equilibrium was upset when the population of the unit was 60 instead of the 40 to 45 it has now been limited to.

This smaller population of patients still complained in many of the interviews of the lack of privacy in the open dormitories, however. Despite the fact that some degree of privacy is possible through performing activities at different times, for example, or using the hospital grounds, it is likely that the withdrawal of patients to their beds reflects psychological constraints on their behaviour.

It is often suggested by the staff that the 'open plan encourages interaction'. Reference to Table 2A indicates a

high degree of 'talk' or interaction in the unit (20.82%).
This characterizes the staff's behaviour and the staff rooms
more than the other areas however. It may be that in reality the dormitories are, to some extent, ambiguous spaces
neither public nor private which tend to mitigate against
interaction or a wider range of behaviour. Support for
this argument is to be found in the mapping studies of
Ittelson et al (1970b). They found that in general in the
psychiatric hospitals they looked at, the smaller the room
(i.e. with the smallest number of patients) the wider the
distribution of activity types. Isolated passive behaviour
rose regularly with the 'size' of bedroom.

Table 2A: Percentage of different activities throughout the
unit (Refer to Table 1)

ACTIVITIES

20.82	5.10	3.79	6.80	3.78	11.65	
Total 100% 3.90	15.51	1.20	8.78	7.83	4.82	6.02

Table 2B: Overall use of different areas of the unit
expressed as percentage

AREAS West End Dormitory	East End Dormitory	Dining Room	West End Lounge	East End Lounge	Front Office	Staff Office	Corridor near Staff Office
W.Do	E.Do	Di	W	E	Fr	St.O	C
12.85	16.22	14.94	20.96	9.14	2.58	5.35	2.90

	Side Rooms	Sluice and Boot Rooms	Night Stations	Treatment Room	Staff Room	Washing Areas and Toilet	Kitchen
	Si	Slu	Ni	Tr	St	W	K
Total 100%	0.96	3.65	0.07	0.21	2.20	3.19	4.82

Lack of activity

The low percentage in Table 2A of certain activities such as games (5.10%), reading (6.80%), or sitting-active behaviour (4.82%) compared with activities such as television watching (15.51%) reflects a number of constraints at work. These include psychological constraints as well as organizational restrictions and the limited provision for small group activities within the building mentioned by some people interviewed. The "lack of activity and limited responsibility" afforded to patients which Hudson (1976) found characterized the unit has already been referred to. Her results are confirmed in part by the observational study, if one equates her comments with activities such as lying on the beds, television watching and the differences in staff and patient activities. There are other recreational facilities elsewhere in the hospital which the patients are free to use. However, Table 2 confirms that there is a relatively high amount of 'traffic' (7.83%) through the building compared with other activities. This is facilitated by the open plan.

The lack of use of certain parts of the unit (Table 2B) is a reminder that the building is not being used as effectively as it might be. Whilst three of the four side rooms are used irregularly (0.96% of the total building use), the staff contend that they are useful for coping with difficult patients. The night stations (0.07%) appear to be generally redundant. There is other evidence (Sime, 1975) which shows that the empty sluice and boot rooms (3.65%) and the side rooms, are rated by patients and staff as the most unsatisfactory and 'institutional' areas of the unit. The night stations and sluice rooms might be considered as the areas which characterize most clearly the architect's original intentions to provide facilities suitable for lower grade subnormal patients. It is not surprising, therefore, that there is some redundancy here.

SOME FINAL CONSIDERATIONS

It is characteristic of a study of this kind that it is easier to point to aspects of the behaviour in the unit which are therapeutically counter-productive rather than those that are valuable. The "relaxed and permissive atmosphere about the unit, which is appreciated by most patients" (Hudson, 1976, p.69) has received no mention.

Two further features of the unit are worthy of mention: (a) its relation to the rest of the subnormal hospital, and

(b) the group therapy. Considering the effect of the unit's location on the patients' attitudes and activities, first, it is apparent that their freedom of movement in the hospital grounds, particularly in the summer months when the present study was carried out, reduced the number of people to be found within the building itself at any one time. While some of the patients interviewed criticised the setting, the hospital does provide a number of recreational and work facilities which are beneficial in terms of the unit's aims. Thus, there are considered by the consultant psychiatrist to be positive advantages in the patients being able to see and mix with others who are 'worse off' than themselves elsewhere in the hospital.

From a brief consideration of the unit's background it is apparent that there is strong association of the building with treatment principles at variance with those of custodial institutions in general. This is a positive factor in dealing with the patients. Despite the therapeutic advantages of being able to use the hospital grounds, however, the patients inevitably feel certain more insidious institutional constraints on their individual activities. It is clear that the building and hospital setting act as an important mediator in interactions between the patients and staff.

A second important therapeutic activity in the unit, the group therapy, has not been considered since it did not occur during the observational study. This activity normally takes place in the lounges. As visiting staff and nurses who participate in groups indicated in their interviews, areas such as the side rooms and dormitories are less conducive to relaxed discussion either because of "bare, cramped conditions" or their "association" with other activities. The lounges, though generally preferred for group therapy, were criticised for being too large, open and subject to interruptions or distractions from people "passing through".

The medical model

While the building itself has provided many positive features for a forensic unit, there is some indication that the layout may have had an inhibitory effect. The notion that the unit is not functioning at an optimal level, a stringent criterion for any therapeutic environment, has already been indicated by the patterns of activity. These reflect the unit's partial adoption of the 'medical model' encouraged by the present design, with its emphasis on 'observation' of the patient activities and a division between staff and patient areas. In this way the degree to which it has been possible to achieve a primary aim, the establishment of a 'mutual support system between staff and patients', has been reduced. To some degree the 'ease of observation' afforded by the design has been replaced by a 'surveillance' model where staff leave staff areas to see what patients are doing, rather than to spend time mixing with them in their own areas.

This medical model characterises many psychiatric and subnormal hospital buildings. Bettelheim (1974) has criticised the fact that hospital buildings for the physically sick still serve as models for mental institutions referring to the 'medical analogy' which bears down on the imagination of the architect and planners of buildings. Seager (1972) echoes this. He points out, for example, that unlike the physically ill patient, the psychiatric patient "is usually up and about and therefore requires to fill his day with some positive activity". For the forensic patient this is equally the case.

Examining the relative merits of the open plan as opposed to a more compartmentalised design it is clear that as the open plan is considered by many patients and staff to be the antithesis of the prison cell it may be symbolically valuable. On the other hand it may deny or limit an individual's personal freedom to perform particular private or small group activities of therapeutic value. Both staff and patients complained in general about the 'lack of privacy', though there was considered to be rather more privacy in the staff areas (except for the staff office) than anywhere else (Sime, 1975). Thus one might question the need for ease of observation perpetuated by the present design.

Physical and organisational changes

The fact that a number of the areas of the unit are hardly used but have not been rearranged or adapted to foster particular activities in line with the therapeutic aims, is perhaps surprising. It was suggested in interviews with staff and patients that quiet or reading rooms, games, visiting and counselling rooms might be incorporated into the building setting. Differences in opinion between staff over the possible function of certain rooms, as well as administrative restrictions and the apparent ease with which people are able to adapt themselves to an environment, all appear to have limited changes.

Future plans

Plans are now afoot to introduce some modifications to the unit and, if possible, to monitor these changes. The symmetrical layout means that the division of one dormitory into 4 to 6 bedded areas and single rooms could be compared with the existing layout at the other end.

The question of how best to maintain a degree of personal freedom within 'peripheral' walls (where the patients are restricted from going outside a building), is one which is now of direct concern in the design of the proposed medium security units for potentially dangerous 'inadequate' offenders (Butler Committee, 1974). In this case the need for a balance between custodial and therapeutic aims is clearer than for the Prentice Unit itself. One such closed 30 bedded unit is currently being planned for the same campus, to work in conjunction with the open Prentice Unit in the future (Sime and King, 1974). The problems characterising the original locked Dart Ward led this hospital to a general policy of unlocking its doors, indicating that if patients in the Prentice Unit were not allowed to use the hospital grounds, it is possible that the open plan design would go much further to minimise personal freedom inside the building than it does at present.

SUMMARY

To summarise the main points raised in the chapter, it has been shown that:

1. The physical environment of a therapeutic (in this case forensic) unit both reflects and influences its overall aims and the functioning of its social organisation. The physical aspects of institutions are rarely considered in any detail in social studies. The findings presented in this chapter suggest that they should be.

2. The nature of the hospital model adopted in a physical design is crucial, since it helps to facilitate patterns of activity which may or may not be appropriate to the therapeutic aims of the unit. The adoption of an existing 'medical' model and open plan design by the forensic unit considered, has not avoided some of the organisational features of a custodial institution. These may have made it easier to contain patients, but have detracted in part from therapeutic aims.

3. The characteristic division of the psychiatric hospital building layout into staff and patient areas, limiting inter-action between the two groups, is perpetuated when the architect adopts existing hospital building models. The therapeutic principles need to be established more explicitly in terms of the activities desired. If the physical environment is not incorporated into the general framework of the therapeutic model, a therapeutic environment is unlikely to be operating at its full potential. This is a conclusion which would benefit from further refinement and testing across a range of institutional settings.

REFERENCES

BETTELHEIM, B. (1974) A home for the heart, Thames and
Hudson, London.

BUTLER COMMITTEE (1974) Report on mentally abnormal
offenders, HMSO (Command No. 5698), London.

CLARK, D. H. (1974) Social therapy in psychiatry, J. Aronson,
New York, also in Penguin books.

CLARKE, B. V. G. and MARTIN, D. N. (1975) "A study of
absconding and its implications for the residential
treatment of delinquents", in Varieties of residential
experience, Tizard et al (see below) Ch.11, pp.249-274.

FRANKENBERG, R. and MILLHAM, S. (1976) Some findings from
material supplied by the Prentice Unit, Dartington
Social Research Unit, February (unpublished).

GOFFMAN, E. (1961) Asylums: Essays on the social situation
of mental patients and other inmates, Doubleday, New
York; Aldine, Chicago.

HUDSON, E. (1976) Prentice Villa. A unit for treatment of
personality disorders, B.Phil. Social Work Dissertation,
Exeter University (unpublished).

ITTELSON, W. H., RIVLIN, L. G. and PROSHANSKY, H. M. (1970a)
"The use of behavioural maps in environmental psychology",
in Proshansky et al, Environmental Psychology, Holt,
Rinehart and Winston, New York, 65, pp.658-668.

ITTELSON, W. H., PROSHANSKY, H. M. and RIVLIN, L. G. (1970b)
"The environmental psychology of the psychiatric ward",
in Proshansky et al (ibid), 43, pp.419-439.

LECOMPTE, W. F. (1972) "Behaviour settings: The structure
of the treatment environment", in Environmental Design,
Research and Practice, EDRA THREE, ed. J. Mitchel,
University of California.

MINISTRY OF HEALTH (1964) Hospital Building Note 32, HMSO, June.

RIVLIN, L. G. and WOLFE, M. (1972) "The early history of a psychiatric hospital for children: Expectations and reality", Environment and Behaviour, 4 (7), March, pp.33-72.

SEAGER, C. P. (1972) Psychiatry and architecture: Review of literature, The Society of Clinical Psychiatrists.

SIME, D. A. and EASBY, F. P. D. (1973) The development of forensic services in Devon, Devon Area Health Authority Memorandum.

SIME, D. A. and KING, D. A. (1974) A regional security unit, Devon Area Health Authority, December.

SIME, J. D. (1975) "A psychological analysis of the Prentice Unit, Langdon Hospital, Devon, M.Sc. Dissertation, University of Surrey (unpublished).

TIZARD, J., SINCLAIR, I. and CLARKE, R. V. G. (1975) Varieties of residential experience, Routledge and Kegan Paul, London and Boston.

Mental Patients and Nurses Rate Habitability

ROBERT SOMMER AND BONNIE KROLL

INTRODUCTION

In response to civil lawsuits, American courts have been taking a closer look at the conditions in state institutions. It used to be that the courts lost interest once a person entered an institution unless some obvious scandal was exposed and an official was charged with a specific wrongdoing. Now the courts recognize that people keep their civil rights even when they come within the jurisdiction of a state facility. The interest of the courts is focused on three issues: (1) due process, (2) humane conditions, and (3) entitlement to treatment. It is the second of these issues, humane conditions, that is of most relevance to environmental psychology.

While one can find earlier court decisions dealing with the mental hospital environment, particularly for patients in restraint or isolation, Wyatt v. Stickney in 1971 is generally regarded as the landmark decision in this area. The court not only decreed Ricky Wyatt's right to treatment in decent surroundings, it spelled out a set of explicit environmental standards in which physical facilities were expected to make "a positive contribution to the efficient attainment of the treatment goals of the hospital" (Ennis and Siegel, 1973). This has led to a concern with habitability as one of the major quality-of-life issues in environmental psychology. Habitability refers to the suitability of an area for its occupants and includes such dimensions as lighting, noise level, crowding, cleanliness, attractiveness, etc. While most courts have been content to use general phrases such as 'adequate and sufficient', several have applied more operational and specific definitions of environmental adequacy, particularly when local

conditions deviate too greatly from community standards.
At the Belchertown (Mass.) State Hospital, the court directed
a specific sum of money to be spent on architectural improvements.

Environmental psychologists are in a unique position
to contribute to the movement for environmental quality in
mental hospitals. For a variety of fortuitous reasons,
much of the early research in environmental psychology took
place in mental hospitals. Most of this, however, followed
a scientific rather than an evaluative model, for example,
Esser (1965) and Ittelson et al (1970). Architecturally-
minded investigators, following a programming model, concentrated on obtaining the informed opinions of hospital administrators and staff. Rarely was any direct comparison made
between the views of patients and staff. The schism underscored the fact that these were two separate social systems
in the hospital, with clearly circumscribed and largely
separate orbits. Even when patients and nurses inhabited
the same ward, they occupied different parts of it. The
situation is even more extreme in the case of psychologists,
psychiatrists, social workers, and other specialists who
appeared on the ward only for brief intervals and rarely if
ever entered sleeping areas, patient dining areas, toilets,
showers, and portions of the lounge, dayroom, and yard.
Numerous studies have documented the tendency of ward staff
to cluster around the nurses' station and other staff areas
(Deane, 1961; Sommer and Ross, 1958). Generally a staff
member found in a patient-dominated area is in transit and
will remain there only for brief periods. Even those employees assigned to direct patient care are not likely to have
first-hand experience with many aspects of the ward environment, including the showers and toilets of the patients'
bathroom (since the staff generally have their own toilets)
or with the comfort of the beds or with the food served to
patients. Because patients and staff tend to occupy different parts of the hospital and use them differently, there
is no reason to assume that their views of the environment
based on their actual experiences should be identical.

Sociologist William Deane, who lived as a patient on a
ward for a week, stated that many parts of the hospital
appeared different to him during his stay. "This is in no
sense a perceptual distortion", he explained. "It is rather
a condition of seeing things through a different set of eyes
which has the effect of making the familiar appear unfamiliar". There is also a good deal of evidence that perception
of all kinds is affected by the duration of stimulation.
Extended viewing makes a bright colour appear duller and an
unusual colour pattern less startling. Katz (1931) found

that short stay patients preferred warm colours such as red and yellow from the short wave end of the spectrum, whereas long stay patients preferred the cooler blues and greens at the other end of the spectrum. Little is known of the sensory adaptation made by patients who have spent years in a drab institutional environment. The slow tempo and drab sensory aspects of the institutional environment undoubtedly have some role in the shock inmates feel when going outside for the first time (Sommer, 1974). Many experience dizziness and nausea during the first trip outside.

In the mid-1970s, the legal situation regarding the environmental conditions of California's state hospital patients had not reached the point of specific court directives. There was, however, the feeling among state officials that this was only a matter of time unless remedial action were taken quickly. Pressures for environmental changes were coming from other directions as well. The U.S. Department of Health, Education, and Welfare (HEW) was threatening to cut off funds for patients in state mental hospitals who received federal payments if suitable accommodations were not provided for them. HEW insisted on conformity with its own standards for hospital environment. Unfortunately, these differed in significant ways from those of the Joint Committee for the Accreditation of Hospitals (JCAH) and also differed from various state regulations. One code for psychiatric facilities defined appropriate privacy as no more than eight beds per room, another code twelve beds, and still another no more than four beds per room. Wyatt v. Stickney in Alabama had specified a maximum of six patients in multi-bed rooms. The confusion about which environmental changes need to be made in which order was an impediment to remedial action. Many of the changes required by HEW, such as partitioned sleeping areas for small numbers of patients, would be exceedingly expensive if implemented on a large scale, and thus drain money away from educational and therapeutic programmes.

This paper will discuss a team effort to make some sense out of the conflicting standards and poorly defined priorities affecting mental hospital construction and renovation. California legislators felt frustrated in considering requests for physical improvements on a piecemeal basis. Every year there would be a request for $1 million for improving the heating system of Hospital A, a request for $3 million to air condition six buildings at Hospital C, a half million dollars to improve the roofing on two buildings at Hospital D, and so on. Advocates of community treatment believed this money would be better spent on local services rather than in improving the large state hospitals. It is

noteworthy that half of the California state hospitals that
had been operating two decades earlier, had already been
closed and their patients placed in the community. To provide some guidance to the state legislature, a major architectural office was hired as the prime consultant and they in
turn hired several subcontractors in areas such as structural
engineering, food and laundry services, health planning, and
habitability. The inclusion of habitability was a direct
outcome of the numerous court decisions on the issue. This
part of the project was assigned to a social scientist (RS)
to handle. He in turn enlisted the aid of an associate (BK)
and several graduate students. The social scientists then
became consultants on the larger project, contractually
similar in role and responsibility to the other consultants.

THE TASK

The task assigned us was to learn something of the suitability of the present hospital environment for patients and
staff and to make recommendations for needed improvements.
These recommendations, it should be realized, would be conveyed to the prime contractor and not directly to the hospital or the state authorities. Because of the incredibly
tight deadline, we would not be able to employ time-consuming
procedures. If we wanted to be useful to the other members
of the team, including the structural engineers and the
architects doing the fire-life safety assessments, we had
to have our information collected and analysed in several
weeks and our recommendations available shortly after that.
Such a timetable is bizarre to anyone accustomed to the
leisurely pace of academe, but it is standard operating
procedure in architectural practice. We opted, therefore,
for an environmental survey since this is probably the fast-
est method of generating a large amount of standardized data.
Fortunately, the subject of mental hospitals was a familiar
one to us, and we already had available a basic environmental
questionnaire. It had to be modified, or course, to suit
the particular institutions, but it was not necessary to
spend great amounts of time developing and pre-testing a
totally new instrument. We also had available rating scales
used in previous investigations of mental hospital environment (Osmond, 1975; Vail, 1966).

Two mental hospitals were selected by state officials
as containing most of the architectural characteristics in
which they were interested. Hospital A had large barn-like
buildings that housed mostly mentally ill patients, but also
several wards of mentally retarded patients. The second
hospital contained cottage-style residences for retarded

patients. The different architectural characteristics of the two hospitals, as well as the patient population, necessitated two separate surveys. The questionnaire consisted of two open-ended questions asking the respondent what he or she liked most and least about the ward, and then to rate various environmental characteristics on a three point scale (good/OK/poor), and to elaborate on any items considered inadequate. The questions were directed to the four major areas of the ward - the dayroom, sleeping areas, dining areas, and toilets. Space was provided at the end for any additional comments. The questionnaires were supplemented by lengthy interviews with various ward staff and administrators as well as observations and evaluations by the interviewers themselves. The final assessment of each ward was a composite of the questionnaire responses from the nurses, interviews or questionnaires collected from patients, and the researcher's own observations.

Although 1,058 staff and patients were surveyed, one should not be misled by this figure into believing that this is anything more than two case studies, one of each hospital. Thus, particular results such as the adequacy of ventilation in the sleeping areas, for example, which was of primary interest to the project team, will be of less interest to outside readers than the meaning of those findings and their relevance for other places and people. We will therefore refrain from including the detailed tabulations which were done ward-by-ward and building-by-building. We do not believe that many readers would be terribly interested in the opinions held by the staff about the lighting in Cottage A. Such information was the primary concern of the other team members in making decisions about the retention, elimination, or renovation of Cottage A.

As on previous projects, we wrote two reports. Copies of the final report containing the detailed recommendations, including the cost estimates for suggested improvements, are on file with the Department of Health, State of California, Sacramento, California, USA. The second, presented here, is a more general outline of the methods and general findings and their implications for other settings. On other projects we have seen the frustration of designers, interested in specific findings who are presented only with general sociological conclusions or when a general audience is presented with an incredibly tedious and detailed assessment of environmental features. The solution, we believe, is for the environmental researcher to write two reports - the first for internal use by project staff, and the second for a general audience.

SURVEY RESULTS: HOSPITAL A

Hospital A, the second oldest mental institution in the state, was founded in 1865. Most of the buildings are quite large, reflecting the period of a decade ago when the institution contained over 4,500 patients. Today the resident population consists of 1,726 mentally ill adults and 371 mentally retarded adults and children. Questionnaires were obtained from 677 staff representing all building types and wards. Individual interviews were conducted with 55 patients. approximately 10 from each of the 5 major architectural types of buildings. The questionnaires were distributed by the hospital administration, filled out anonymously by staff, and placed in a large envelope in the ward office, to be collected by one of the researchers. The patient interviews were done individually and took approximately one hour per interview. Patients who had been selected on the basis of staff assessment as being articulate and cooperative, were informed of the purpose of the interviews and asked about their willingness to participate. There were very few refusals and patients were very cooperative. The term 'nurse' in this article is used in a generic sense to refer to all nursing staff, including registered nurses, psychiatric technicians, and nurses' aides. All the nursing staff surveyed were direct line-of-care employees.

Nursing staff viewed the interior areas largely from the standpoint of their responsibilities. Their opinions of the environment were inextricably tied to the number of staff available relative to the number of residents. A cottage might work well with six staff, but if only three staff were available, it would be a disaster. Good surveillance became more necessary as the number of staff decreased. With a generous allocation of nurses, nooks and crannies and partitioned areas where patients could get privacy, were considered desirable. With a small staff, these same partitioned areas created surveillance problems. Essentially any discussion of the adequacy of space must take into account the number of staff and patients and the particular activities that occur. Since it is often difficult to predict occupancy rates too far in advance, this poses a great challenge to the designer. Not only will a hospital suitable for North London work poorly in South London, but it may not even work well in North London if the number of resident patients doubles or the number of staff is reduced by a third. The interdependence between a physical structure and the social system must be recognized. This is another reason why awards for distinguished buildings should not be given without post-occupancy evaluation. There is no such entity as a good psychiatric hospital (or good bank or good office building) without regard to its environmental/social context.

Staff frequently complained about the lack of separate toilets on the wards, a lack of staff sinks, and individual offices. When staff lounges were available, they were popular but usually too small. We found many nursing stations that were of inadequate size, hot and stuffy. Occasionally work surfaces were lacking and there was no room to sit down. Staff felt that inadequate working conditions produced fatigue and irritability among nurses.

Most staff had formed opinions of the patient-dominated areas, either based on the nurses' own experiences or statements made by patients. Aesthetic qualities of the units generally were poor. Bare concrete walls, a lack of drapes, pictures, and other wall decorations, drab colours with no designs, and tacky institutional furnishings were prevalent. Patios, courtyards, and porches were very popular when usable, but often a shortage of staff limited patient access to them. The size of most dayrooms, dormitories, and dining halls is considered far too large with high noise levels resulting from conflicting uses.

Ward size was generally much too large for effective programming. Residents in wards containing 40 to 70 patients could easily be lost track of for short periods, even though they were on the ward. Surveillance of such a large number of residents was a problem for staff, and tolerating the crowding, confusion, and noise a problem for patients. There was a shortage of rooms appropriate for group therapy and activities, so that groups sometimes convened in shower rooms, toilet areas, or corners of dayrooms or dormitories where they were subjected to constant interruption and a general absence of privacy.

A lack of resident privacy in the sleeping areas and bathrooms was one of the worst features of the hospital as a whole. There were no wards where bathing or toilet areas were adequate. Lack of shower curtains and toilet doors were the predominant complaints, along with a bathroom layout which features tubs, open toilets, and showers in direct line of sight with the bathroom entrance. Supervision needs conflicted directly with the patients' needs for privacy. Residents felt extremely uncomfortable under these conditions, and many were unable to satisfy needs for hygiene with so little privacy. Most residents slept in large dormitories lined with rows of beds interspersed with unlockable lockers. Dining rooms were the most successful interior areas on

campus, with all units reporting conditions adequate or
better. There were practically no odour problems, and the
dining areas were clean, and table arrangements and decorations were satisfactory. A recommendation of our report
was that dining areas should be opened up during the rest
of the day for other activities. Often their use was restricted specifically to dining.

It was felt that some of the deficiencies of the living
units could be remedied by getting more residents to outside
activities. Staff often complained that they were limited
in their ability to escort patients outside the wards and
for transporting them longer distances. Many of the problems
encountered in implementing therapy programmes and providing
a reasonably aesthetic comfortable environment stem from the
age of the buildings and their design for custodial use.
These large barrack-like wards were designed for corraling
large groups of people in one area and having them stay
there. Such spaces do nothing to promote the interpersonal
interaction needed in modern milieu therapy, nor do they
encourage or even permit the everyday activities similar to
those found in the outside world.

SURVEY RESULTS: HOSPITAL B

This hospital was first established in 1891 on a 1,700
acre estate chosen for its attractive natural setting, its
mild climate, abundant water supply, and convenient access
to railway lines. The present population consists of 1,966
mentally retarded children and adults who live in 43 buildings,
most of which are cottage style. Questionnaires were collected from 312 nursing staff, including at least 5 nurses from
each residential unit. Individual interviews were held with
19 high functioning retardates, all of whom were picked by
staff as able to participate in the survey.

Hospital B contained highly diverse buildings both with
respect to size, age, complexity, and adequacy of maintenance
efforts. A common element cutting across building and residence characteristics is that most structures were designed
for grouping of 50 or more occupants. This conflicts with
the scale of social unit now thought to be optimal for most
retarded patients - a 'family unit' of 10 to 12 residents.
The social identity of family units in the large, undifferentiated spaces was maintained through room dividers and
furniture arrangements with less than optimal success. The
consequent confusion of traffic through a family area, because other families are leaving the building, for example,
interrupted programming. There was a general lack of small
and medium sized rooms.

Some exterior yards were green and attractively planted but were not always accessible to severely retarded patients or those in fragile health. Other courtyards were of asphalt and completely lacked any natural features such as grass or trees. The staff generally felt that daily access to the out-doors was of great benefit to residents. The climate at both hospitals permitted this virtually year-round. For those patients inside the building, windows were often too high for an outside view, so that residents confined to bed could only see the sky and tops of trees, and residents sitting lacked any outside view.

The smaller buildings of Hospital B, compared to Hospital A, created more attractive living spaces. Most of the dayrooms were adequate as interaction spaces, and satisfactory in terms of physical characteristics, especially natural light. Many of the sleeping areas were large and barrack-like with little provision for privacy or adequate ventilation. Large numbers of incontinent residents or those not thoroughly habit-trained created odour problems in the dormitories. As in Hospital A, the dining areas were satisfactory or excellent, with many units having homey table arrangements, curtains, and decorations. The lack of privacy was the worst aspect of bath and toilet areas. In some cottages there were toilets without seats in long open rooms that also served as corridors for travel. If a single word could characterize staff goals for patient living areas, it would be homelike. This feeling seems much more pronounced among the staff in the cottages of Hospital B than in the long barrack-like structures of Hospital A. This reflects the different programme responsibilities of the two institutions - Hospital A for the mentally ill seeing its mission as therapeutic and modelling itself after the general hospital, and B seeing its role as primarily custodial/educational modelling itself after a home or private residence.

Interviews with 19 high-functioning residents in 5 different living units indicated that the most important environmental attribute from their standpoint was the quality of staff, followed closely by the amount of bedroom privacy. Private or semi-private rooms were highly prized and taken as evidence of capability in self-help skills by those residents who were sensitive to the privacy issue. Other residents, however, did not see anything wrong with large dormitories and unpartitioned toilets. This was taken as the normal state of things. In both A and B, the staff were more critical than patients regarding the aesthetic qualities of the environment. The responses of the patients were most useful in regards to specific items overlooked by staff, such as the adequacy of the mirrors for combing hair, size

of the sinks, temperature variations in the showers, spacing
of beds for wheelchair patients who needed extra room to
manoeuvre during bedmaking, the height of light switches etc.

CONCLUSION

In general, the staff was far more critical than residents regarding the quality of the living space. Many patients
passively accepted what was obviously deficient from a staff
viewpoint. This was particularly true of long stay patients
who remembered the hospital as it had been when it was terribly overcrowded. Both hospitals were today more overcon-
centrated rather than overcrowded. The buildings and living
units contained too many people even though the amount of
space per inmate was adequate. Patients who remembered a
ward as it had been when three times the number of patients
occupied the same amount of space and used the same number
of toilets and showers could not help but express appreciation
at the improvement. Other patients had been in the hospital
so long that they lost any basis for making comparisons and
accepted the drab conditions without complaint. Previously
we found such patients resisting efforts to make wards more
homelike by, for example, moving the chair away from the
wall and placing it with others in conversational arrangements. Patients who had been in the hospital shorter periods
of time were generally more specific and more critical in
their responses (Sommer, unpublished). Patients' opinions
were invaluable in regards to specific items of concern to
them. We feel that straightforward questions to patients,
even those who are moderately retarded or senile, can produce
a considerable amount of valuable information about the ward
environment that could not or would not be obtained in any
other way.

We finished our research with some ambivalence about
the value of the questionnaire approach in this sort of
situation. Although it allowed us to collect a great deal
of information quickly and economically, it rarely provided
anything beyond what was noticed by the observers in their
visits to the units. The ratings of some nurses were often
too specific or too general. This is an inherent defect in
a questionnaire with fixed answers. To have used open-ended
questions would have presented an impossible task in coding
and tabulation and still, we fear, some of the responses
would have been too specific and others too general. Perhaps
there is no feasible solution when one is making an environmental assessment of 500 or more different spaces, each with
its own characteristics. It is relatively easy to present
this on a room-by-room basis, for example speaking of the

showers in Wright Cottage or the ventilation in the sleeping area in Ward B-6. These are the sorts of statements of direct concern to architects and administrators.

The most frustrating aspects for us were the tight deadline and consultant role. The questions were given to us by the client who then proceeded to use only that portion of the information that was felt to be relevant. Certain issues such as the possible closing of additional state hospitals were off-limits to us. The final report was restricted to the kinds of changes that were needed and their potential cost without reference to the effectiveness of the institutions. Even so, we believe that our information on habitability improved the final report if only as a counterweight to the recommendations of the other consultants. For example, the structural consultants were very impressed by the durability and structural integrity of several of the concrete barracks in Hospital A. From an engineering standpoint, these buildings would probably last forever. The engineers were likewise extremely critical of the small wooden and stucco cottages, some which had previously been staff residences, which were used for special programmes. From a structural standpoint these buildings did not meet hospital construction codes. Our recommendation based on habitability were the reverse of those based on durability. In the opinions of both staff and patients, the huge concrete barracks were the worst buildings, and the cottages the best. Rather than tearing down the cottages and putting a great deal of money into removating the huge barracks, we felt it would be preferable to change the state regulations to make provision for residential buildings that did not meet the standards of a general medical hospital, and to tear down the oversized concrete monstrosities. We were also able to make recommendations based on existing social science research on privacy and partitioning. Given the defined missions of the mental hospital in terms of custody and therapy, there is an inherent conflict between privacy and surveillance needs. This can only be handled on a ward-to-ward basis with reference to staffing patterns, kinds of patients, and programme. Hospital A has already been faced with several lawsuits from parents of patients who escaped and subsequently injured themselves. There are strong institutional pressures to avoid taking risks and thereby subordinate privacy to surveillance needs. One task of behavioural scientists is to get privacy (and sociability) needs back into the programme.

Environmental surveys can be done quickly and economically in most sorts of institutions and have therapeutic value in their own right. Some survey instruments, such as

those developed by Osmond and Vail, are intended primarily
to make ward staff aware of the possibilities for environmental improvement. Asking nurses, for example, whether
there is a large calendar visible in the dayroom or whether
patients' storage space for photographs of their loved ones,
has considerable value in raising consciousness. Patients,
too, appreciate being asked for their opinions. Occupational
therapist Susan Cross (1960), who interviewed patients to
find out the colours of craft materials they preferred, mentioned how pleased they were to be asked for their opinions.
Many believed that no one cared what they thought. Katherine
Vavra (1956), found very positive feelings towards an environmental survey she conducted in a tuberculosis sanitorium.
An environmental inventory reinforces the patient's individuality because it demonstrates that his or her opinions
matter. Surveys counteract the habituation to the physical
environment that occurs in any institutional setting.

POST SCRIPT

Six months after our final report was turned in,
Hospital A was stripped of its accreditation by the Joint
Commission on the Accreditation of Hospitals. Most of the
deficiencies were environmental, such as the absence of
partitions and doors in bathrooms and toilets, a lack of
privacy in sleeping facilities and showers, undesirable
odours, a lack of opportunity to be outdoors, and a shortage
of individual storage space. The Deputy Director of the
Health Department commented that the denial "is part of the
changing scene in hospitals. We used to have 100 bed wards,
now we're down to 30 and 50. They are pushing us to upgrade
the physical qualities and staffing in the hospitals.
Hospital A", he added, "is probably one of the better hospitals in the state system".

REFERENCES

CROSS, S. D. (1960) "Color preferences of older patients", Canadian Journal of Occupational Therapy, 27, pp.9-12.

DEANE, W. (1961) "The reactions of a non-patient to a stay on a mental hospital ward", Psychiatry, 24, p.67.

ENNIS, BRUCE, and SIEGAL, L. (1973) The rights of mental patients, Avon Books, New York.

ESSER, A. H. et al (1965) "Territoriality of patients on a research ward", in J. Wortis (ed.) Recent Advances in Biological Psychiatry, Vol.8, Plenum Press, New York.

ITTELSON, W. H., PROSHANSKY, H. M., and RIVLIN, L. G. (1970) "The environmental psychology of the psychiatric ward", in H. M. Proshansky et al (eds.) Environmental Psychology, Holt, Rinehart, and Winston, New York.

KATZ, S. E. (1931) "Color preferences in the insane", Journal of Abnormal and Social Psychology, 26, pp.203-209.

OSMOND, H. (1975) Ward environment scale, Bryce Hospital, Tuscaloosa, Alabama.

SOMMER, R. and ROSS, H. F. (1958) "Social interaction on a geriatrics ward", International Journal of Social Psychiatry, 4, pp.128-133.

SOMMER, R. (1961) "Reactions of long and short-stay mental patients", unpublished manuscript.

SOMMER, R. (1974) Tight Spaces, Prentice-Hall, Englewood Cliffs.

VAIL, D. (1966) Dehumanization and the Institutional Career, Charles C. Thomas, Springfield.

VAVRA, C. E. and RAINBOTH, E. D. (1956) "A patient's opinion survey at Firland Sanitorium", Public Health Reports, 71, pp.351-359.

Environmental Psychology in Psychiatric Hospital Settings

CHARLES J. HOLAHAN

HISTORICAL PERSPECTIVES

Until recently human beings have tended to ignore the impact of environmental alterations on themselves (Proshansky, Ittelson, and Rivlin, 1970). Behavioural scientists, for example, have viewed the environment as the passive background of behaviour which is determined by programming that people carry around within themselves, rather than as a dynamic shaper of human events (Barker, 1965). Until a decade ago, scientific investigation of person-environment systems was restricted to a handful of designers and scientists. Since that time, however, scientists of varied backgrounds have joined the developing group of investigators in this area, and the hybrid discipline of environmental design research is emerging (Sanoff and Cohn, 1970).

The environmental sciences are at present without a theoretical foundation (Canter, 1970; Hufschmidt, 1966; Proshansky et al, 1970). In lieu of theory, the following defining characteristics have been advanced by Proshansky et al (1970) as a functional definition of the environmental sciences: they are concerned with the built environment, they have emerged from pressing social problems, they are multidisciplinary in nature, they include the study of human beings as a vital part of every problem.

Izumi (1965) offers a diagram useful in understanding the meshing of human and nonhuman components in the architectural fabric. Imagine a rectangle (Figure 1) to represent environmental design as related to buildings, with a diagonal separating the human and nonhuman factors. At the left, are buildings designed essentially to contain objects, machinery, equipment and other inanimate objects. At the right, are

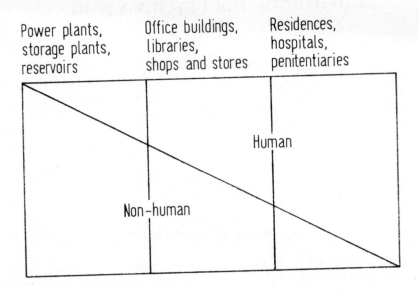

Figure 1: The field of design (Izumi, 1965)

buildings designed solely to contain human beings, as for example, nursing homes, penitentiaries, psychiatric hospitals, and housing in general. Between these extremes are buildings used to contain both people and objects in varying proportions. These include libraries, laboratories, stores, and offices. As we move from left to right in the diagram, the evaluation of buildings becomes progressively more weighted toward performance as a social setting and against visually aesthetic properties (Deasy, 1970; Sommer, 1969). Nevertheless, many contemporary buildings fail to achieve behavioural requirements, because of all the types of information on which architectural decisions rely, the category of activity is often the most deficient (Watson, 1970).

All of these considerations point to the importance of examining the design of hospitals in the light of man's psychological and social needs. It is indeed ironic that of all building forms, the hospital is one of the most resistant to change; "visual patterns persist like vestigial characteristics long after their functional needs have changed" (Lindheim, 1966). A number of research studies concerned with investigating hospital environments have adopted a model approximating that described by Barker (1965). These studies typically have compared behaviour over macroscopic settings in the hospital which are a complex of physical, social, and cultural factors. The studies

of LeCompte and Willems (1970) and of Rosengren and DeVault
(1963) in medical hospitals are in this tradition, as are
the studies of psychiatric wards by Moos (1968) and Raush,
Dittmann, and Taylor (1959) and Raush, Farbman, and Llewellyn
(1960).

Other studies in hospital environments have selected,
at the level of independent variable, specific features of
physical design and experimentally abstracted these physical
components from the total macroscopic setting. The need
for this type of research has been pointed to by Field (1971)
and Watson (1970), who have underscored the need for the
physical design of hospitals to meet the requirements of
their dynamic activity systems. The physical environment
of psychiatric hospitals has been the focus of vigorous
criticism (Agron, 1970; Osmond, 1957; Sivadon, 1970). Osmond
(1957) describes a well known British mental hospital which
"welcomes its new arrivals in a richly painted and gilded
hall. Among the intertwining leaves covering the walls,
goblin-like creatures are concealed. Sometimes a whole head
can be seen, sometimes only an eye gleams malevolently at
the new arrival". A number of authors have stressed the
need for environmental research dealing with the therapeutic
and antitherapeutic effects of psychiatric hospital settings
(Bailey, 1966; Foley and Lacy, 1967); Griffin, Mauritzen,
and Kasmar, 1969; Stainbrook, 1966).

Significant first steps have been made by researchers
concerned with investigating the physical environment of
psychiatric hospitals in relation to patient behaviour. A
continuing series of environmental studies in psychiatric
hospital settings has been conducted over the last decade
by researchers in the Environmental Psychology Program of
the City University of New York. These investigators have
used "behavioral maps" (Ittelson, Rivlin, and Proshansky,
1970) to relate patient behaviour to specific physical locations in the hospital setting. Ittelson, Proshansky, and
Rivlin (1970b) reported significantly more passive, withdrawn behaviour by psychiatric patients in both a city and
a state hospital compared to patients in a private hospital.
These same investigators (1970a, 1970c) also found an increase in passive, withdrawn behaviour in hospital bedrooms
as a function of increasing occupancy. Rivlin, Proshansky,
and Ittelson (1969) have conducted one of the few studies
where the behavioural effects of an experimentally induced
change in a psychiatric ward setting have been systematically observed.

A number of investigators have pointed to the perceptual ambiguity and distortion induced by the physical design

of many psychiatric hospitals. Spivack (1967) has testified
to the auditory and visual perceptual distortions caused by
the elongated tunnels and corridors prevalent in many psychiatric facilities. Izumi (1965) and Osmond (1957, 1959)
have discussed the fearful reactions to perceptual ambiguity
experienced by schizophrenic patients.

Kasmar, Griffin, and Mauritzen (1968) examined the
impact of interview rooms of contrasting aesthetic appeal
on the mood and perception of outpatients at the U.C.L.A.
Neuropsychiatric Institute. Sivadon (1970) has reported
favourable therapeutic success at the Marcel Riviere Institute
in France, where the architecture, size, and spatial relationship of buildings, in addition to the structure of
outdoor grounds have been designed in terms of specific
therapeutic objectives.

Although psychiatric patients spend considerable time
in dayroom settings (Rivlin et al, 1969), there is evidence
to indicate that these settings tend to inhibit social and
functional behaviours while coercing passive isolation
(Harmatz, Mendelsohn, and Glassman, 1970; Ittelson et al,
1970; Mendelsohn, 1969; Sommer, 1969; Sommer and Ross, 1958).
Two environmental studies have underscored the relationship
between seating patterns in hospital dayrooms and patients'
social behaviour. In a Saskatchewan hospital, Sommer and
Ross (1958) altered the seating arrangement from an unsocial
to a social pattern. Chairs which had previously been
arranged shoulder-to-shoulder along the walls of the dayroom
were moved closer together in small groups around tables.
With the new furniture arrangement, social interactions
among patients were doubled in frequency. In a New York
City hospital, Rivlin et al (1969) converted the seating in
an unsocial corner of a solarium on a psychiatric ward to a
more social arrangement. The reorganization created increases in conversation between occupants of this part of the
room besides increasing overall use of the area.

Some researchers (Hall, 1969; Osmond, 1957, 1959;
Sommer, 1969) have distinguished between spaces which facilitate social interaction and spaces which inhibit such
interaction. Osmond (1957, 1959) defined as "sociopetal",
spaces which encourage or foster the growth of stable interpersonal relationships. Osmond lists as examples of sociopetal spaces, tepees, igloos, and Zulu kraals, while railway
stations, jails, hotels, and hospitals are typically sociofugal spaces. Sommer (1967) has noted that the isolation
of schizophrenics in mental hospitals can be increased by
sociofugal settings which restrict social contact, or reduced

by sociopetal settings which facilitate social behaviour.
Hall (1969) has indicated that sociopetal space is not uni-
versally good. He contends that the most desirable space
is flexible space where individuals may or may not be
socially involved depending on the occasion.

CASE STUDY I: SEATING PATTERNS AND THERAPEUTIC OBJECTIVES[1]

The purpose of this study was to clarify further the
effects of contrasting dayroom seating arrangements on the
behaviour of psychiatric patients. An experimental hospital
dayroom was arranged to afford a setting where the effects
of specific and controlled manipulations in seating could
be observed on small groups of patients. In Sommer and
Ross's study, for example, although the results were attributed to the change in seating patterns, a number of other
simultaneous changes in the ward environment confound the
clarity of this interpretation. Confounding factors included
the introduction of an occupational therapist and an improvement in ward attractiveness during the sociopetal phase of
the study, along with social pressure from nurses to sit in
the sociopetal arrangement. In the present study each of
these possible confounding factors was removed by manipulating seating patterns in a controlled experimental dayroom.
It was hypothesized that a dayroom characterized by sociofugal seating would demonstrate less social interaction than
would settings characterized by sociopetal or mixed seating.

Procedure

Subjects were 120 hospitalized male psychiatric patients
recruited from four unlocked wards at a Veterans Administration Hospital. Patients were randomly assigned to 20 six-
member groups, and five groups were randomly assigned to each
of four experimental conditions. The experimental conditions
were as follows: sociofugal - chairs were arranged shoulder-
to shoulder along walls of the room; sociopetal - chairs were
arranged around a small table in the middle of the room; free-
patients were told to arrange the chairs themselves in any
manner they wished. The four experimental conditions are
depicted visually in Figure 2.

Chairs were arranged in their experimentally defined
position before each session, and patients in all except the
Free condition were told not to rearrange the furniture.
Each group participated in one experimental condition for a
45-minute session. An observer was located in an extended
area of the room, six feet from the nearest chair. In a

218

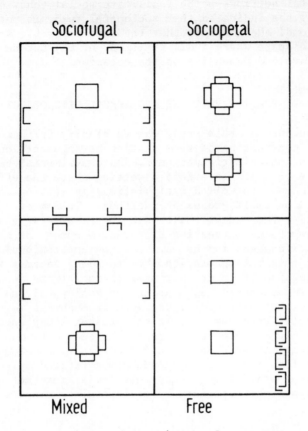

Figure 2:   Seating patterns in the four treatments

time sampling procedure, each subject's behaviour was recorded at 75-second intervals.   The behaviour categories used
in the study are based on the work of Hunter et al (1962)
and Ittelson, Rivlin and Proshansky (1970).   Two additional
measures were collected after the behavioural observations
were completed.   First each subject was given a map of the
room and told to draw eight chairs to show his preferred
room arrangement.   Second, the following unobtrusive measures
were taken: (1) cigarette butts left in the room were coun-
ted; (2) the quantity of coffee consumed was measured;
(3) the length of time patients remained in the experimental
setting after the session had ended was recorded.

Results

Table 1 shows the mean number of behaviours per group
under each behaviour category for the four experimental

conditions. There was significantly less social interaction in the sociofugal setting than in either the sociopetal setting (t=2.60, df=16, p<.01, one-tailed test) or the mixed setting (t=2.35, df=16, p<.025, one-tailed test). A surprising finding was the very low level of social behaviour in the free setting.

Table 1: Mean group behavioural scores

Behaviour categories	Experimental conditions			
	Sociopetal	Mixed	Sociofugal	Free
Conversation	61.8	40.8	32.0	16.8
Verbal games	14.6	9.6	.6	5.0
Other verbal	1.2	.4	.6	.4
Total verbal	77.6	50.8	33.2	22.2
Nonverbal games	32.2	30.6	4.2	18.0
Other nonverbal	.6	.8	.6	0.0
Total nonverbal	32.8	31.4	4.8	18.0
Total social	110.4	82.2	38.0	40.2
Nonsocial active	47.2	55.8	53.2	55.4
Nonsocial passive	77.8	87.6	123.2	120.6

The overall differences between settings in verbal interaction were statistically significant at the .025 level (F=4.31, df=3/16), with the mean verbal interaction for the sociopetal and mixed conditions significantly greater than that for the sociofugal and free conditions (F=3.56, df=3/16, p<.025). The treatment effect for conversation was statistically significant at the .025 level (F=3.40, df=3/16), with the mean conversation for the sociopetal and mixed conditions again significantly greater than that for the sociofugal and free conditions.

Discussion

These findings in a controlled setting lend strong support to the position (Hall, 1969; Osmond, 1957; Sommer,

1969) that sociopetal spaces facilitate social interaction, while sociofugal spaces inhibit such interaction. The present results also support the findings of Sommer and Ross (1958) in an actual hospital dayroom. A consistent difference between settings showed the sociopetal and mixed settings to be more social than the sociofugal and free settings. Patients' seating choices in the free and mixed settings indicated that patients preferred sociopetal to sociofugal seating. The low level of social participation in the free setting was probably in part a function of past training in the hospital environment. Psychiatric patients have been consistently trained to be "outer-directed", while training for self-directed social encounter and environmental management has been greatly neglected.

There were important qualitative differences between the types of conversation which developed in the sociopetal and the sociofugal settings. The sociopetal conversation was characterized by an evenness of flow, a great deal of involvement, and a high level of psychological closeness and intimacy. Typical topics of conversation included: home visits, personal problems, service experiences, and finances. The sociofugal conversation, in contrast, proceeded in a sporadic manner and typically lacked spontaneity and involvement. Topics of discussion were rarely personal or intimate, and typically involved food, baseball, dayroom activities, and past acquaintances in the hospital.

These findings may be translated into the following specific practical terms. A greater amount of conversation and psychologically closer and more intimate conversation will occur in sociopetal dayroom seating arrangements than in sociofugal ones. Also, multi-person conversations are more likely to develop in sociopetal settings. Allowing patients to arrange their own dayroom furniture appears unprofitable without prior training in self-directed environmental management. Past tendencies to ignore the behavioural impact of physical settings and to perceive hospital environments as unalterable should not be allowed to present an insurmountable obstacle to productive and therapeutic environmental change.

CASE STUDY II: THE PROCESS OF LARGE-SCALE CHANGE[2]

Earlier research investigating the relationships between physical environment and psychopathology in treatment settings has generally precluded large-scale manipulation of the environment. Recently, however, we were able to plan, finance, and direct the extensive remodelling of a psychiatric ward in a New York City hospital. This research was made possible by a grant from the U.S. Public Health Service to William Ittelson. The initial planning of the remodelling changes was carried out by Willian Ittelson and Susan Saegert.

Procedure

The remodelling was based on the preferences and dis-satisfactions expressed by patients and staff in interviews and on our observations of behaviour on the ward. The design was intended to encourage successful social interaction and to discourage withdrawal. Before remodelling, the walls on the ward were dirty and peeling, and were marred by scrib-bling that was rarely cleaned. Furniture on the ward was old, worn, and rather uncomfortable. The remodelling was designed to (a) qualitatively improve the ward atmosphere, and (b) achieve a number of specific behavioural effects. The changes concerned with improving ward atmosphere inclu-ded repainting the ward and the addition of new furniture. A range of bright colours was chosen for the repainting, and attractive, modern furniture was added in the dayrooms and bedrooms. A number of additional changes on the ward were concerned with creating areas on the ward which afforded a range of social options - from a high degree of privacy to a high level of social participation. A private sector was created in the bedrooms by installing six-foot-high partitions, creating a number of two-bed sections in each dormitory. A table and two comfortable chairs were installed in a screened-off area of each bedroom to allow for private conversations. Small group interaction was encouraged in one dayroom where new tables and chairs were arranged in small social groupings. Larger group socializing could occur at large tables in the dining room.

There was an opportunity to employ an experimental con-trol in this hospital since a second admissions ward was available which was identical to the remodelled ward before change. Twenty-five patients were randomly selected for observation on each of the two wards. Experimental measures were initiated six months after the remodelling was completed to allow sufficient time for enduring ward routines to become established. Experimental measures were collected in an identical manner on the two wards during a simultaneous five-week period. Five patients were studied per week on each ward. Observation sessions of seventy-five minutes were conducted on both the morning and afternoon of Mondays and Thursdays. A time sampling procedure was used in which an instantaneous recording of each patient's behaviour was performed at five-minute intervals.

Behavioural results

We predicted that after the remodelling, patients on the remodelled ward would engage in more social behaviour and be less passive and withdrawn than patients on the unchanged control ward. These hypotheses were supported. Table 2 depicts mean behaviour per patient in each behaviour category on the remodelled and control wards. The mean difference between the two wards in total social interaction was statistically significant at the .05 level with a directional test (t=1.78, df=40). The mean difference between the two wards in total isolated passive behaviour was statistically significant at the .05 level with a directional test (t=1.84, df=40). The higher level of total social behaviour on the remodelled ward occurred across all areas on the ward.

Table 2: Mean behaviour per S in each behaviour category on the remodelled and control wards

	Behaviour categories	Remodelled ward	Control ward
SOCIAL	Social with patients	7.3	5.1
	Social with staff	3.8	2.6
	Social with visitors	3.2	1.1
	TOTAL SOCIAL	14.3	8.8
NON-SOCIAL	Engaged in activity	9.5	9.9
	Observing activity	5.6	3.5
	Walking	6.7	8.3
	TOTAL NON-SOCIAL ACTIVE	21.8	21.7
	Isolated passive awake	7.1	11.5
	Isolated passive sleeping	11.8	15.8
	TOTAL ISOLATED PASSIVE	18.9	27.3

Temporal phases of environmental change

We have observed four time-ordered phases in the psychological impact of the remodelling - petrification, unfreezing, resistance, and personalization.

Petrification

One of the most compelling phenomena we observed on first entering the ward was a petrification of the ward environment. Over time, the established structure of the physical environment had become rigidly set, with both staff and patients viewing these established patterns as practically unalterable. This petrification pervaded the entire physical environment, including standard ward design, the usual types and arrangements of furnishings, and typical colour preferences. Sommer and Ross (1958) have referred to this phenomenon as "institutional sanctity". Whatever environmental change did occur within the ward occurred in a "patch-work" fashion. Such change is characteristically unsystematic and narrowly pragmatic in that it responds to immediate needs without deliberating long-term impacts. Patch-work change gravitates toward the traditional mould, as when new furniture delivered to the ward during the remodelling was immediately arranged by staff in the previous unsocial manner along the walls of the dayroom.

Unfreezing

Kurt Lewin (1947) wrote that in order for permanent change to be achieved, the change agent must first unfreeze the old level of performance. In the remodelling study, we realized that productive environmental change was possible only after the prevailing philosophy on non-change had been altered. This involved replacing the existing body of expectations that militated against change in the ward system, by new expectations that viewed change as both possible and desirable. Lippitt, Watson, and Westley (1958) propose the following factors as essential in the unfreezing process: (a) individuals in the setting must be aware of existing problems; and (b) they must have confidence in the possibility of a more desirable state of affairs.

Ward staff did not at first consider the lethargic behavioural style on the ward as a therapeutic problem. Also, after having experienced repeated frustrations in initiating change through the hospital bureaucracy, staff evidenced only minimal faith in the prospect of real change. We thus accepted as our first task instilling problem aware-

ness among ward staff. To this end we met with represent-
atives from all ward staff levels in a series of informal
sessions to discuss potential ward needs. At these meetings
we presented in a simplified summary form data from a pilot
behavioural mapping as feedback demonstrating the markedly
passive and unsocial quality of daily life on the ward.
Since this data clashed sharply with the staff's expectation
that the ward provide an acceptable social atmosphere for
patients, it helped to achieve problem awareness, along with
a desire for improvement. Our second challenge was to establish confidence in the possibility of change. For this
purpose we used an initial change - delivering new equipment
to the game room - which was easily effected, highly visible,
and likely to produce immediate behavioural effects.

After these initial efforts, we were able to proceed
with a cooperative planning effort, which involved agreeing
on specific remodelling features and selecting appropriate
contractors. This does not convey that unfreezing was completed through our initial strategy. Despite the fact that
our funds were available to execute the changes, we worked
throughout the planning period against recurring pessimism,
bureaucratic entanglements, embedded competitiveness between
staff groups, and a diffusion of decision-making responsibility in the hospital. During this period, we played a
facilitative role with ward staff, sharing encouragement
and listening openly to fears and grievances. Though we
operated within the established power structure in the hospital, we made a concerted effort to keep all levels of
staff interested and involved in all phases of planning.

Resistance

Although resistance to change operates covertly even
during the pre-change period, it surfaces as real change
begins and the implications of change, which was previously
thought impossible, are suddenly felt or imagined. Simply
initiating environmental change in the psychiatric hospital
is not enough, since the impact of change can be undone
behaviourally, administratively, or politically. The period
during and immediately after the actual renovation of the
admitting ward was not the emotionally positive phase we
anticipated. Instead this period was characterized by a
generalized feeling of tension on the part of the ward staff,
and by a sense of reserve, coldness, and emotional distance
in ward staff's behaviour toward us. In part this behaviour
probably reflected the staff's perception of us as "outsiders", who despite the best intentions could never fully
appreciate the insider's intimate knowledge of ward life.
In addition, we were especially impressed by how much change

itself was feared and how unwilling staff members were to take personal responsibility for change. Resistance was particularly evident when role changes were involved, as when an environmental change implied a new staff behaviour toward patients. Both the administrative structure and peer pressure militated against innovation on the part of staff members. For example, when the ward activity therapist proposed a new treatment philosophy during the change period, he was reprimanded by a supervisor for "overstepping his bounds".

A clear example of resistance developed around our effort to install partitions in the large dormitories of the admitting ward to create a more private atmosphere for patients in the bedrooms. Although all parties had agreed verbally to the plan in advance, the nursing staff abruptly decided against it on the day carpenters arrived to implement the changes. They complained that partitions would make it impossible to survey the bedrooms from the hall as was previously possible. The nursing staff harassed the unwitting carpenters to such an extent that they quit the job, and refused to return until we contacted them directly. A compromise was reached by lowering a number of smaller partitions to facilitate surveillance. However, we later discovered that for two weeks after the changes the evening staff had not assigned any patients to the new bedrooms, choosing instead to put patients in alcoves and the hallway! In retrospect, this behaviour is understandable in the light of jealousies between evening and day staff of which we had been unaware, and of our own failure to adequately involve the evening staff in the change process.

Personalization

Resistance to environmental change is inversely related to the degree of control people feel in producing that change. Resistance decreases dramatically as people are able to personalize the changes in their surroundings. This is a critical phase in the change process. Effective environmental change does not occur outside of the people in a particular setting; these individuals are themselves involved in and changed by the change process. To a great extent we encouraged such personalization in the ward renovation, but much of this phenomenon operated outside of our control and in excess of our expectations.

An open-house party on the newly completed ward was initiated and organized by ward staff themselves, and served as a clear public notice that the changes were their changes. Also, staff extended the planned changes by adding touches of their own, as when the nursing assistants made curtains for the dayroom and dining room with money they raised on the ward. An interesting aspect of personalization was also observed in the behaviour of patients on the post-change ward. Whereas before renovation almost no personalization of space by patients occurred on the ward, after the change personal articles, such as books, magazines, towels, powder, and flowers, were observed on the window ledges of the newly partitioned bedrooms. Interestingly, openness to change at one level provided an impetus for a simultaneous openness to change at other levels. As the remodelling was being completed, ward staff began meeting on their own initiative to discuss for the first time the development of a ward treatment philosophy. As a result of these meetings, staff members began to perceive the previously ignored needs, concerns, and frustrations of members of other staff groups.

UNDERSTANDING ENVIRONMENTAL CHANGE

It is important to consider the psychological processes involved in translating change in the physical environment into change at the level of the ward social system. Two factors appear to be of significance. First, new expectations were developed by the physical changes. The improved physical environment implied a greater interest, hope, and involvement in a therapeutic philosophy. Thus, ward staff felt expected to play a stronger role in therapeutic planning and programming. The feeling of increased self-importance ward staff perceived as a result of the environmental improvements was significant in this process. Second, the remodelling task itself demanded a new level of competence on the part of ward staff at all levels. Ward staff were forced to demonstrate and practice a range of highly competent behaviours in planning for the changes, from selecting colour preferences to determining an optimum number of beds for the new bedrooms. Competence was also demanded from ward staff in executing the changes, from arranging new furniture in the dayroom to keeping painters and patients from interfering in one another's activities. We encouraged this process across all levels of staff by soliciting, facilitating, and legitimizing input from all staff groups throughout the change process.

The increased feeling of competence and effectance on the part of ward staff learned in the environmental change process generalized naturally to other role behaviours involving therapeutic planning, interpersonal staff relations, and more healthy contacts with patients. The enhanced therapeutic atmosphere on the ward after the remodelling can be explained in terms of the more competent role behaviour of ward staff rather than as a result of a more positive attitude toward patients. From the beginning ward staff perceived the remodelling in terms of personal comfort and ego enhancement rather than as an effort to create a better atmosphere for patients. In fact, one impact of the remodelling was to accelerate staff expectations for career advancement. For example, on the postchange ward, one nurse sought an administrative position, an activity therapist decided to earn a graduate degree, and an aide planned to enter nursing school. Even the ward janitors became so involved in the new ward's upkeep that their work was held up as a model in the hospital's housekeeping unit.

The role of the environmental change agent

The reader may question how the change process presented here might be compared with the type of change discussed in the organizational change literature. We would propose that the two change processes are quite similar. Essentially both represent structural changes in the social system of an organization initiated through change efforts by an out-side agent. The systemic shift from resistance to person-alization discussed here bears an important similarity to current views of organizational change. The traditional organizational change model accepted the point of view of the change agent as rational, and assumed the resister's view to be irrational. A more current view enhances the role of the resister as vital to the system's survival, and underscores the value of the change agent's making positive use of this energy during the change process (Klein, 1969). Our discussion of resistance has stressed our original ego-centric view as frustrated change agents. The personaliz-ation process represented the involvement in the change process of positive adaptive capacities within the system which we were forced to respond to and to make use of. In addition, many of the basic social psychological issues involved in environmental change are identical to those considered in the organizational change literature, such as establishing organizational goals, clarifying group decision-making, improving the communication network, and resolving intergroup conflict.

FOOTNOTES

[1] An extended version of this study is available in the Journal of Abnormal Psychology, 1972, 80, pp.115-124.

[2] An extended version of this study is available in Human Relations, 1976, 29, pp.153-166.

228

REFERENCES

AGRON, G. (1971) "Some observations on behaviour in institutional settings", Environment and Behaviour, 3, pp.103-114.

BAILEY, R. (1966) "Needed: optimum social design criteria", The Modern Hospital, 106, pp.101-103.

BARKER, R. G. (1965) "Explorations in ecological psychology", American Psychologist, 20, pp.1-14.

CANTER, D. (1970) "The place of architectural psychology: a consideration of some findings", in J. Archea and C. Eastman (eds.) Proceedings of the 2nd Annual Environmental Design Research Association Conference, Carnegie-Mellon University, Pittsburgh.

DEASY, C. M. (1970) "When architects consult people", Psychology Today, 3, pp.54-57 and pp.78-79.

FIELD, H. H. (1971) "The environmental design implications of a changing health care system", paper presented at Environment and Cognition Conference, City University of New York, Graduate Center, June.

FOLEY, A. R. and LACY, B. N. (1967) "On the need for inter-personal collaboration: psychiatry and architecture", American Journal of Psychiatry, 123, pp.1013-1018.

GRIFFIN, W. V., MAURITZEN, J. H. and KASMAR, J. V. (1969) "The psychological aspects of the architectural environment: a review", American Journal of Psychiatry, 125, pp.93-98.

HALL, E. T. (1969) The Hidden Dimension, Doubleday, New York.

HARMATZ, M., MENDELSOHN, R., and GLASSMAN, M. (1970)
"Naturalistic observation of hospitalized schizophrenic
patients", unpublished manuscript, University of
Massachusetts.

HUFSCHMIDT, M. (1966) "A summary of environmental planning",
The American Behavioural Scientist, 10, p.628.

ITTELSON, W. H., PROSHANSKY, H. M., and RIVLIN, L. G. (1970a)
"A study of bedroom use on two psychiatric wards",
Hospital and Community Psychiatry, 21, pp.25-28.

ITTELSON, W. H., PROSHANSKY, H. M., and RIVLIN, L. G. (1970b)
"The environmental psychology of the psychiatric ward",
in H. M. Proshansky, W. H. Ittelson, and L. G. Rivlin
(eds.) Environmental psychology: man and his physical
setting, Holt, Rinehart, and Winston, New York.

ITTELSON, W. H., PROSHANSKY, H. M., and RIVLIN, L. G. (1970c)
"Bedroom size and social interaction of the psychiatric
ward", Environment and Behaviour, 2, pp.255-270.

ITTELSON, W. H., RIVLIN, L. G., and PROSHANSKY, H. M. (1970)
"The use of behavioural maps in environmental psychology",
in H. M. Proshansky, W. H. Ittelson, and L. G. Rivlin
(eds.) Environmental psychology: man and his physical
setting, Holt, Rinehart, and Winston, New York.

IZUMI, K. (1965) "Psychosocial phenomena and building
design", Building Research, 2, pp.9-11.

KASMAR, J. V., GRIFFIN, W. V. and MAURITZEN, J. H. (1968)
"Effect of environmental surroundings on outpatients'
mood and perception of psychiatrists", Journal of
Consulting and Clinical Psychology, 32, pp.223-226.

LECOMPTE, W. and WILLEMS, E. (1970) "Ecological analysis
of a hospital: location dependencies in the behaviour
of staff and patients", in J. Archea and C. Eastman
(eds.) Proceedings of the 2nd Annual Environmental
Design Research Association Conference, Carnegie-Mellon
University, Pittsburgh.

LEWIN, K. (1947) "Frontiers in group dynamics", Human Relations, 1, pp.5-41.

LINDHEIM, R. (1966) "Factors which determine hospital design", American Journal of Public Health, 56, pp.1668-1675.

LIPPITT, R., WATSON, J., and WESTLEY, B. (1958) The dynamics of planned change: a comparative study of principles and techniques, Harcourt, Brace and World.

MENDELSOHN, R. (1969) "The relationship between length of hospitalization and ward behaviour in schizophrenic patients", unpublished Ph.D. dissertation, University of Massachusetts.

MOOS, R. H. (1968) "Situational analysis of a therapeutic community milieu", Journal of Abnormal Psychology, 73, pp.49-61.

OSMOND, H. (1957) "Function as the basis of psychiatric ward design", Mental Hospitals, 8, pp.23-30.

OSMOND, H. (1959) "The relationship between architect and psychiatrist", in C. Goshen (ed.) Psychiatric Architecture, American Psychiatric Association.

PROSHANSKY, H. M., ITTELSON, W. H., and RIVLIN, L. G. (eds.) (1970) Environmental psychology: man and his physical setting, introduction, Holt, Rinehart and Winston, New York.

RAUSH, H. L., DITTMANN, A. T., and TAYLOR, T. J. (1959) "Person, setting and change in social interaction", Human Relations, 12, pp.361-377.

RAUSH, H. L., FARBMAN, I., and LLEWELLYN, L. G. (1960) "Person, setting and change in social interaction. II: a normal-control study", Human Relations, 13, pp.305-331.

RIVLIN, L., PROSHANSKY, H. M., and ITTELSON, W. H. (1969) "Change in psychiatric ward design and patient behaviour: an experimental study", unpublished manuscript, City University of New York.

ROSENGREN, W. R., and DEVAULT, S. (1963) "The sociology of time and space in an obstetrical hospital", in E. Freidson (ed.) The Hospital in Modern Society, Free Press, New York.

SANOFF, H., and COHN, S. (1970) Preface, in H. Sanoff and S. Cohn (eds.) Proceedings of the 1st Annual Environmental Design Research Association Conference, North Carolina State University, Raleigh.

SIVADON, P. (1970) "Space as experienced: Therapeutic implications", in H. M. Proshansky, W. H. Ittelson, and L. G. Rivlin (eds.) Environmental Psychology: Man and his physical setting, Holt, Rinehart, and Winston, New York.

SOMMER, R. (1967) "Small group ecology", Psychological Bulletin, 67, pp.145-152.

SOMMER, R. (1969) Personal space: The behavioral basis of design, Prentice-Hall, Englewood Cliffs, New Jersey.

SOMMER, R. and ROSS, H. (1958) "Social interaction on a geriatrics ward", International Journal of Social Psychiatry, 4, pp.128-133.

SPIVACK, M. (1967) "Sensory distortions in tunnels and corridors", Hospital and Community Psychiatry, 18, pp.24-30.

STAINBROOK, E. (1966) "Architects not only design hospitals; they also design patient behavior", The Modern Hospital, 106, p.100.

WATSON, D. (1970) "Modeling the activity system", in H. Sanoff and S. Cohn (eds.) Proceedings of the 1st Annual Environmental Design Research Association Conference, North Carolina State University, Raleigh.

Therapeutic Environments
for the Aged

POWELL LAWTON

INTRODUCTION

For much of this century solutions to the 'problem' of
the aged have been sought through somewhat grudging and
condescending attempts to be kind to older people in traditional social-welfare style. The problem was thus defined
in terms of the elderly alone. As the average lifespan has
become extended, however, the proportion of the populations
of industrialized societies that reaches the magic age of
65 has correspondingly increased. Social programmes for the
aged such as retirement and health-care benefits account
for an increasingly greater percentage of all public expenditures; all indications point to a further increase at
least until the year 2000. Thus relatively suddenly the
problem of the aged has been recognized as a societal problem that involves all of us: all of us pay for the programmes
now and most of us will be future beneficiaries.

An important sector of programming for the aged involves
the design of environments that may be thought of as supportive or therapeutic in the broadest sense: community planning,
transportation, housing, and institutions. Much of the
planning for such environments is done either intuitively
or on the basis of experience gained in contexts other than
those that are concerned with the specific needs of the
elderly. When the need reaches critical proportions, it is
all too easy to justify less than completely rational planning. The purpose of this chapter is to demonstrate that
there is, in fact, more knowledge available than is now
being utilized, and that environments for the elderly may
be produced with better result when this knowledge is incorporated into the planning and design process.

233

Sources of design-relevant knowledge

Since both gerontology and environmental psychology are relative newcomers to contemporary scientific inquiry, there are more than the usual number of gaps in firmly established knowledge. Nonetheless, there has been considerable research activity in the environmental psychology of later life, whose results will be reviewed. A clearly preferable basis for design decisions is conclusions from empirical research that directly test the effect of an environmental feature on the behaviour or the psychological state of older people. A second choice that in the absence of such on-target research is frequently forced on the designer is the application of knowledge about the potential user that may be extrapolated into design decisions even though the knowledge itself relates more to the individual than to the environment. Careful consideration of the characteristics of older people (and subgroups of the elderly) and their needs significantly increases the likelihood that the product will be supportive, as compared to the unthinking importation of design principles of known relevance only to younger people. Thus, some highlights of gerontological knowledge of possible, but indirect, relevance to environment design will be sketched briefly. The remainder of the presentation will be devoted to the application of both environment-specific and general knowledge in gerontology to typical environmental problem areas.

ENVIRONMENT-RELEVANT KNOWLEDGE ABOUT OLDER PEOPLE

Much of the literature in gerontology has overemphasized the deficits associated with the later years of life and has conveyed the unfortunate impression that massive impairment is characteristic of people 65 and over. Careful study of the body of knowledge reveals, however, that many fewer negative changes are associated with chronological aging in and of itself than is commonly thought. Given good physical health, a comfortable economic position, and a social context that is relatively free of negative stereotypes and 'ageism' (Butler, 1969), an older person will function as well or as poorly as she did during earlier life. Such fortunate exemption from the strains of existence regretably applies to relatively few elderly people, however. In the USA, 80 per cent of the elderly suffer from one or more chronic diseases. Retirement has become increasingly mandatory, and in 1973 the average income of older people was less than half the average income of people of working age (Brotman, 1976). Ample documentation of the prejudicial attitudes of society expressed on both an interpersonal (Bennett and Eckman, 1973) and a social-policy level (Butler, 1975) is at hand. These deprivations, while not the inevitable result of aging, characterize enough older people to warrant our concern with programmes designed to compensate for these deficits.

For the purpose of this chapter, a therapeutic environment is seen as any physical or organizational structure whose purpose is to elevate the functioning of an older person in a way that counteracts any of the deficits that are statistically associated with the process of growing old in a Western social context. Elsewhere the author has suggested that environmental barriers and facilitators become increasingly critical to the well-being of the older person as his competence is diminished by biological, social, or economic factors - the 'environmental docility hypothesis' (Lawton, 1970a). The positive aspect of this hypothesis lies in the probability that small increments in environmental quality may result in a disproportionate increase in the quality of life for those with such deficits. The deficits to be discussed are those for which environmental intervention seems particularly appropriate.

Physical health and security

As age increases the probability of chronic disease shows a parallel increase, and acute illnesses become more life-threatening. Thus the accessibility of medical care is a much more salient aspect of the environment than for younger people. Needs for safety from fire, accidents, crime, and environmental pollutants are similar to those of people in general, but deficits in health and in the other areas to be described below result in older people's being selectively vulnerable. As a principle of environmental design, proximity to health care, emergency service, and neighbours who can help is desirable, as is increased concern with the design of safety features in all environmental settings.

Sensory processes

Most of the senses show age-related decrements. Since all environmental information comes through the senses, a wide variety of difficulties in apprehending and negotiating the environment may result. Visual problems include a loss of acuity, narrowing of the visual field, slowed accommodation to temporal or spatial changes in illumination,

sensitivity to glare, and some loss of colour differentiation. Hearing becomes less acute, particularly in the
higher frequency range on which speech and other signals
depend for their clarity. Auditory distortion becomes more
of a problem, as does the capacity to filter out extraneous
auditory noise in favour of the focal stimulus. Awareness
of one's body position (kinesthetic sense), of temperature
changes, taste, and smell may in some cases be disturbed.
In addition to the specific reductions in knowledge about
the environment that these sensory changes cause, the outer
world may approach an undifferentiated state that deprives
the older individual of the environmental variation that is
so necessary to a sense of excitement; the need for stimulus
variation has been shown to be a basic human need (Fiske
and Maddi, 1961). Improvement in the negotiability of the
environment may often be achieved by making stimuli clearer.
Some examples may illustrate the great diversity of aids
that may thus be achieved:

- Pedestrian paths should be sharply differentiated
  from vehicular paths.

- Large size lettering with high contrast is desirable
  for signs.

- Stair treads should contrast with risers in colour,
  brightness, and texture.

- Glare from outside light or reflective surfaces
  should be minimized so that detail in less-lighted
  areas may be discerned.

- The intensity of auditory signals (telephone, fire
  alarms) may need to be greater.

- Highly contrasting colour, brightness, and texture
  will enrich the sensory environment; a homogeneous
  field, as deliberately used in so many institutional
  environments, is not only disorienting but also
  depressing.

Cognition

While recent research has tended to confirm that much
of the decline in intellectual capacity that was formerly
presumed to be an essential component of the aging process
is explainable on the basis of factors other than chronological age (Baltes and Labouvie, 1973), many of these
extraneous factors are themselves more prevalent among the

aged, and a few cognitive changes appear to be age-related.
Central nervous-system processing time does seem slower with
age. Complex, unfamiliar, and unpredictable situations may
evoke less adaptive responses, particularly when stress is
high and the time for processing or response is limited.
Learning shows fewest deficits when there is no time pressure
and especially when the older individual can control the
pace at which the learning occurs. While not in any way
characteristic of most older people, cognitive disturbances
resulting from central nervous system pathology have been
estimated to occur in 5 to 10 per cent of the older population, including half or more of those in nursing homes
(National Center for Health Statistics, 1967).

Design principles will thus demand that attention be
paid to enhancing the meaningfulness of the environment,
the simplicity of the messages conveyed, the familiarity of
signals, objects and spaces, and the removal of time constraints on decisions or motor performance. As concrete
illustrations, one might think of:

- Signs designating the function of a building or
  room ('Warden's Office').

- A schematized map of a single underground route,
  rather than a complex map showing all routes.

- Water fixtures either with separate hot and cold
  levers or with clearly designated temperature and
  flow indicators, rather than a single lever that
  must be operated by trial and error.

- Highway signs that programme decisions in a logical
  sequence and with adequate warning (e.g., 'Norwich
  exit 2 miles', followed by 'Left lane for Norwich',
  then, 'Norwich, turn left 500 feet').

Self-Maintaining Behaviour

National surveys of older people in the USA, England,
and Denmark (Shanas et al, 1968) showed that substantial
proportions of older community residents had difficulty in
performing tasks necessary for daily living. For example,
in England, 27 per cent reported difficulty in walking stairs,
15 per cent in washing and bathing, and 10 per cent in
dressing or putting on shoes. While most of these deficits
are secondary to the deficits in health, sensory capacity,
and cognition mentioned above, the self-maintenance skills
have a wide range of variability around the deficit-determined

level of functioning; the amount of functional deficit may be highly dependent on the environmental situation of the individual.

As Perin (1970) has discussed at length, an environment that responds to the behaviour of the individual induces the feeling of competence, which is in turn a major determinant of basic self-esteem. Young people can cope with recalcitrant zippers, cups that cannot be firmly grasped, storage areas that require stooping or the use of a chair to reach, and so on. While all people would be better off with such design improvements, the elderly would be disproportionately benefited.

Meaningful time use

Multiple factors contribute to the lesser engagement of older people in activities that stimulate them: health problems, difficulties in locomotion, a shrinking social world, retirement, low income, the negative attitudes of society, and a lifetime of necessary preoccupation with activities other than the pursuit of leisure. "Too much time on my hands" is a familiar complaint. For example, in a large sample of retirees, only 15 per cent reported having done any 'handiwork', and one per cent any work with 'crafts or collections' on the day prior to an interview (Beyer and Woods, 1963).

Environmental design intervention in the service of meaningful activities will frequently be on a macroenvironmental level, where the object is to decrease the functional distance between the older person and facilities for leisure time pursuits (see discussion below of neighbourhood design and transportation). Other 'pressure points' may be the reduction of barriers to mobility (steps, unsafe pedestrian paths), the planning of physical facilities for such activity in public places (chessboards in parks, an art studio in a community centre) or in residential and institutional environments (card room or auditorium).

Interpersonal relations

One of the most frequent deprivations in old age is the loss of spouse, relatives and friends through death. Widows comprise an increasingly greater proportion of the aged in successive decades; about 34 per cent of the 65 plus population of the USA lives alone or with non-relatives (US Department of Health, Education, and Welfare, 1973). While people who are socially active in earlier life tend to remain active in old age, each of the other deficits noted in this section may constitute a barrier to contact with friends and family. While the 'disengagement theory' (Cumming and Henry, 1961) suggested that it was both normal and conducive to life satisfaction for people to narrow their social worlds as they enter old age and approach death, empirical research suggests that this situation applies to only a minority of the aged (Lowenthal and Boler, 1965). Environmental barriers such as distance, lack of transportation, and unsafe neighbourhoods may prevent many older people from interacting with friends as much as they would like. Others may have difficulty satisfying their needs for privacy in such situations as the sharing of a household with younger family, living with a spouse in small quarters, or in an institution.

Increasing satisfaction with interpersonal relations will thus require, first, the judgment as to whether a target group's opportunities for social contact are being constrained; if so, then planning so as to decrease the functional distance between potential social contacts and the older person should be followed. Second, if social contact might be demanded to a stressful degree of the older person (for example, in an institution), then design decisions that would enhance the opportunity for privacy, while still not constraining sociability, should be sought.

Psychological health

Despite the many potential deficits listed above, older people's outlook on life generally is as positive as that of people of any age, in terms of ideologies, such as avowed 'happiness' (Riley and Foner, 1968). However, when judged by the incidence of pathological conditions such as depression, suicide, or alcoholism, the mental health of the elderly is poorer than that of the younger population (Butler and Lewis, 1973). Many of the negative social attitudes toward aging to which the elderly have been socialized through a lifetime persist as they themselves age, resulting in a poor self-concept. Many will have the expectation that 'senility' will inevitably overtake them and will experience undue anxiety over minor lapses of memory, difficulty in concentration, or the slowing of cognitive and motor processes. Unresponsiveness in the physical environment is often the occasion for an erosion of the feeling of competence, perhaps the most basic of all intrapsychic problems. The maintenance of a state of relative independence is a goal for which older people seem to be willing to make many other sacrifices.

Social attitudes

The environment-relevant aspects of social attitudes
toward aging range far and wide and may be expressed in
policy and planning decisions such as the amount of money
allocated for structures serving the elderly and standards
for building, land use, and so on. The social climate for
the older person may be directly affected by decisions that
control the characteristics of the other people who are in
close physical proximity to the older person, as in the
decision to create age-homogeneous or age-heterogeneous
housing. Generally speaking, the social norms that operate
in most naturally-occurring environments are likely to be
those of the cultural majority, that is, the adult working
population; some important benefits to the elderly may occur
when age-appropriate norms have the chance to become established in an age-dense environment.

DESIGN APPLICATIONS

This section will examine how general knowledge about
the aged and specific research findings in the environmental
psychology of later life may be applied to the design problems of neighbourhoods, transportation, housing, and institutions. More extended treatments of these topics may be
found in Lawton (1975), Lawton, Newcomer and Byerts (1976),
Green et al (1975), and Byerts (1973).

One may well wonder why some of the more obvious design
suggestions are not routinely followed. There are many
explanations for the frequent failure to implement them.
First, all too frequently there is little attention given
to pre-design planning involving communication among designer, client, potential users, and research workers in environmental psychology. Second, costs are often assumed to be
greater if one departs from tradition in order to serve the
specialized needs of a particular user group. This assumption is often unwarranted but not often questioned, nor are
the long term social gains of an initially higher cost considered adequately.

Neighbourhood design

Most neighbourhoods simply grow, rather than being carefully planned. However, enough new neighbourhoods or even
total communities are still being planned to make it worthwhile to consider some of the potential results that might
be expected in an ideally planned neighbourhood. The

infirmities of old age, economic limitations, and in some
cases a simple preference restricting one's social space
result in a greater local dependency of many older people
for their access to goods and services. Thus, planned concentrations of the elderly should be carefully located near
public transportation, senior activity centres, grocery
shopping, drug store, medical and social service facilities.
Research evidence is clear in showing that location of these
facilities within easy walking distance greatly increases
the use of such facilities (Newcomer, 1973).

The question of age-concentration is a perennial issue
in planning. Given the choice, most older people will prefer
to live embedded in a neighbourhood with a normal age range
(Lawton, 1976a). However, a significant minority (estimated
at around 30 per cent in an urban USA sample, Lawton, 1976a)
would actively prefer living among middle-aged and older
adults only. Such people prefer to have few young children
and adolescents in their immediate vicinity as well as to
be able to choose their associates from people who have
shared values, life experiences and social norms. Therefore,
while a new community should provide enough smaller units
scattered throughout the community to satisfy the needs of
the many who wish thus to be integrated, most will also find
people who will actively seek sections or buildings that are
limited to those 55 and over, or 65 and over.

In existing neighbourhoods, opportunities for such planning are fewer. However, the collaboration of urban planners,
welfare administrators, and municipal officials can do much
to increase the livability of existing neighbourhoods. Since
older people tend to live in older and poorer areas, these
neighbourhoods are prime candidates for redesign. In urban
areas of the USA, a major factor in the well-being of the
elderly has been found to be their feeling of personal safety
(Lawton, Nahemow, Yaffe, and Feldman, 1976). Where the local
crime rate is high, attention can be given to the removal of
derelict buildings, street lighting for high-risk areas, the
removal of low shrubbery or undergrowth along pathways used
by the elderly, and the withholding of liquor licences in
areas where the elderly are concentrated.

Locational decisions for medical and social agencies
serving the aged should be based at least partially on their
accessibility to concentrations of the elderly, proximity to
transportation routes, and safety of the neighbourhood.
Risks to the elderly pedestrian may be minimized by longer
timing of automobile traffic signals, large and clear signs,
the provision of pedestrian 'go' signals in both directions
at intersections, and curb cuts for easier crossing by people

unsure of their footing or those using canes and wheelchairs.
Recognition of sensory, motor, and information-processing
deficits thus can lead to many prosthetic design decisions.

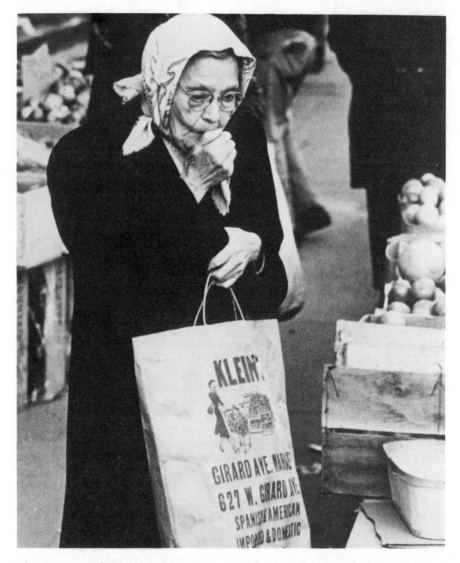

Figure 1: Neighbourhood richness of shopping facilities has
many advantages: exercise, the entertainment of 'window
shopping', and the ability to make frequent trips carrying
small loads. (Photo courtesy of Administration on Aging,
United States Department of Health, Education, and Welfare).

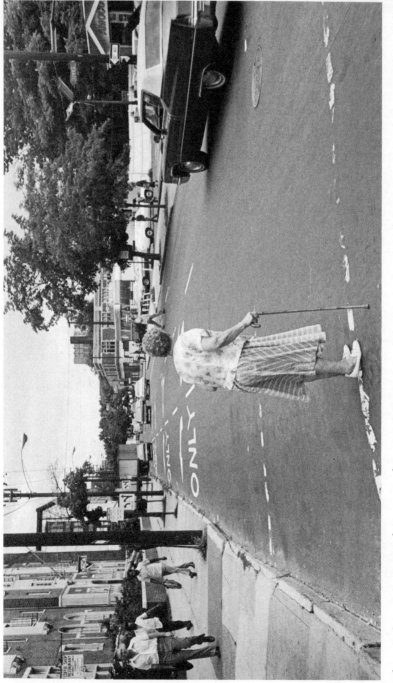

Figure 2: A pedestrian crossing used by many older people requires a pedestrian traffic light. This woman's vigilance is concentrated in the wrong direction for the one-way traffic. (Photo by George Gardner)

Parks are often an important social aspect of the neighbourhood. Byerts (1976) has shown how a favourably located and designed city park can represent an extension of the older person's dwelling. A park border that allows one to sit in a green area while still affording a view of active pedestrian and automobile traffic is a favoured location for the elderly. Park benches with arms to use in arising from them, and of the correct height, depth, and seat slope for the elderly can make park use more gratifying. A 'zone' for the elderly may be encouraged by the provision of facilities for card playing, chess, checkers, shuffleboard, bowling, and so on, as well as safe and clean toilet facilities. As long as seats are provided near children's play areas for the elderly who enjoy this much proximity to the young, the additional development of separate areas for the elderly is to be encouraged. Particularly well used by older people are small 'vest-pocket' parks located near busy urban shopping intersections, where much interesting activity may be observed.

Transportation

While many older people continue to own and drive cars, Carp (1971) has found that this proportion decreases greatly for both biological and economic reasons, and walking and public transportation assume greater importance as modes of transportation. In many cases, public officials are not sensitized to the importance both of routing buses through areas of high concentration of the elderly and of designing the routes so as to include critical resources such as a shopping centre, a medical facility, and a senior recreation centre. The design of public vehicles leaves much to be desired from the viewpoint of the elderly user. The height of the typical bus floor requires higher risers on the steps than is comfortable for many elderly people; not only is mounting a bus unsafe, but this prospect in itself may discourage use of the system. It is possible to design a bus with a lower floor or with a different step arrangement to circumvent this problem. Many existing underground and elevated railway lines are inaccessible because of the lack of alternatives to stairways. Particular attention must be given to making route signs at stops and on vehicles both legible and informative; considerable anxiety may be experienced about getting on the wrong vehicle when the user is unfamiliar with the route, limited in vision, or unable to process the information on destination signs in the necessary time.

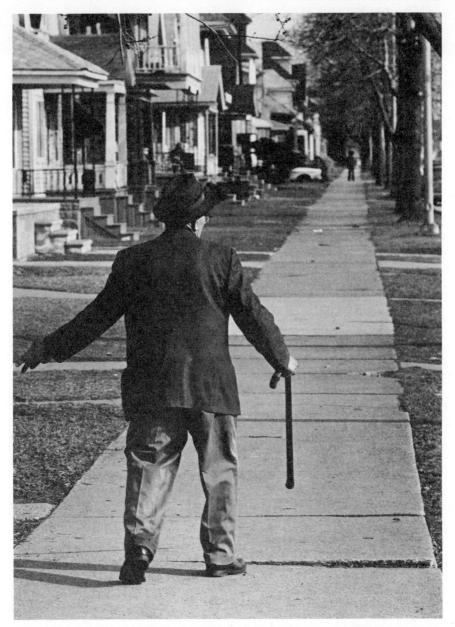

Figure 3: Walking is one of the most frequent forms of transportation. Neighbourhoods with high concentrations of the elderly require special attention to sidewalk maintenance.

Even with careful attention being given to such details, the mass transit system remains relatively inflexible. Thus, a variety of special purpose transportation modes have been developed, including private vehicles driven by volunteers, vans from manufacturers' regular stock, or vehicles designed with special access modes such as hydraulic lift, special seating space arrangements to accommodate wheelchairs, or a 'kneeling' bus whose whole body lowers closer to the street level for mounting and demounting. Service organizations for the elderly will often be better equipped to operate vehicles of varying sizes to run either prescheduled or on-call routes ('dial-a-ride') that will connect elderly users with needed resources. Finally, for those who are homebound, or for clusters of elderly living in resource-poor neighbour-hoods or sparsely settled areas, services may be brought to the people, as in meals-on-wheels, a travelling clinic, or a team of service workers.

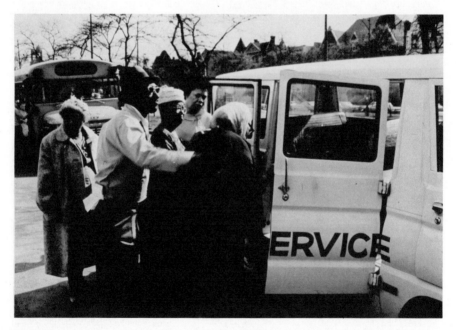

Figure 4: For some older people going to some destinations, personalized transport routes provided by service agencies are required.

In summary, transportation is a vital link to both life-supporting and life-enriching services for older people, and therefore one of the most effective prosthetic interventions

for counteracting many of the deficits associated with aging.
The critical importance of transportation was best illustrated
in research by Ashford and Holloway (1972), who showed that
older people's trip lengths were no different from younger
people's, once a trip had been initiated. In other words,
they availed themselves of the opportunity to use their
greater leisure time, once the barrier to the transportation
opportunity had been overcome. More detailed treatment of
the transportation problems of the elderly may be found in
Golant (1976).

Housing

In the USA, only about three per cent of the aged population lives in housing explicitly built for older people,
and 70 per cent live in homes that they own. By contrast,
a very small proportion of federal expenditures has been
invested in ordinary non-purpose-built housing, and little
of the research literature has dealt with owned or rented
structures in 'normal' communities. While the needs of the
majority have thus been relatively neglected, purpose-built
housing for the elderly is an important phenomenon that has
the capacity to affect the lifestyles of many older people
and is therefore worth extended discussion.

Purpose-built housing for the elderly

Despite the feeling of some critics that project-type
housing ghettoizes the elderly, several research evaluations
have documented the generally favourable effect of planned
housing on its tenants (Carp, 1966; Lawton and Cohen, 1974;
Sherwood et al, 1972). Improvements in housing satisfaction,
social contacts, organizational activity, and general life
satisfaction have been found in rehoused groups as compared
to people who remained in the community. An important aspect
of their satisfaction is the physical improvement in housing
quality that most new tenants experience. Comfort is likely
to increase, but so also are physical security and the feeling of competence. Barriers such as mandatory stairways,
poorly designed dwelling-unit spatial layouts, and excessive
distances to sources of emergency help, are generally lacking
in purpose-built housing. Much security is afforded by the
presence of standard safety features such as an emergency
signalling system, water temperature controls, front door
supervision, grab bars, a night light marking the bathroom,
and so on. Many less obvious design features will make the
performance of everyday tasks of living easier, which in turn

will make the occupant feel more competent and inevitably raise her self-esteem. Some examples are:

- The provision of more storage space than might be thought necessary, since the feeling of maintaining ties to the past is a vital aspect of self-esteem. Lawton (1977) found that satisfaction with storage space was highly related to general satisfaction with purpose-built housing.

- Maximizing the amount of storage space that requires neither stooping low nor reaching too high.

- Full turning radius for wheelchair users in bathroom and kitchen.

- A bathtub with seat and flexible shower hose.

- Full length lighted mirror to encourage continued concern for grooming.

- Dining area and table large enough to enable visitors to be entertained.

- Short hallways or distances to centralized facilities.

- Clear signs to designate important locations or pathways.

At least as important as these security- and competence-inducing features is the capacity of a physical structure to facilitate social relationships among the elderly, which appears to be one of the major reasons for the success of housing projects for the elderly. The basic principle is that spatial design determines whether people's paths will cross in incidental ways, and that such encounters constitute a necessary condition for some kinds of social behaviour. The entrance lobby of a single-entrance building is such a critical nexus, since most tenants must traverse this area repeatedly. Lawton (1970b) found the lobby to be the most used public area of 12 housing estates for the elderly. When conditions permit, this is a highly prized location for sitting, since it allows both the opportunity to interact with others and the equally gratifying experience of watching the behaviour of others and thereby maintaining contact with one's environment. Therefore, the lobby should be relatively large and contain considerable seating space with a view of

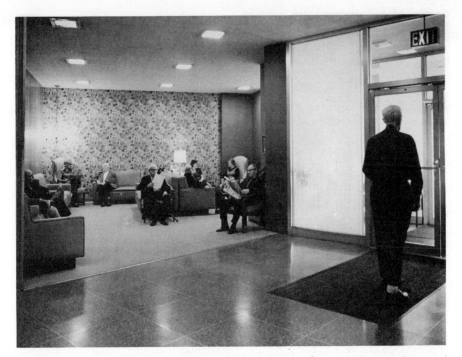

Figure 5: An entrance lobby with a good view of front door traffic is a necessity for the high rise apartment building. (Photo by Sam Nocella, reproduced from Lawton, M. P. Planning and Managing Housing for the Elderly, with permission of Wiley-Interscience, publishers.)

the building entrance, staff offices, and pedestrian pathways. Locating other important spaces near the lobby-elevator-entranceway centre will also increase their accessibility to tenants. Thus, as design constraints allow, staff offices, elevators, and social rooms should be clustered on the ground floor near the centre. Space for more obligatory functions, such as a medical clinic or dining area, can afford to be somewhat more peripherally located. Lawton (1970b) found that outdoor seating oriented toward the building entrance or toward the walkway or the street received the greatest use. Some fixed outdoor seating arrangements may be made to encourage different kinds of social groupings: two benches placed in an L shape form the best orientation for social interaction; three persons on a single bench cannot converse comfortably. Smaller social areas in locations of natural congregation are also useful, as in a laundry room, a waiting room for a medical clinic, or a foyer adjoining a dining area. Small sitting rooms on upper residential floors are infrequently used when no planned activities occur there

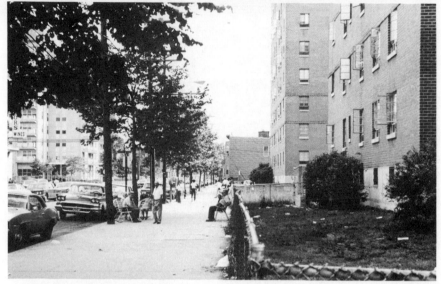

Figure 6: Even where well-designed outdoor seating is not provided, tenants will find a way to socialize where interesting sidewalk activity occurs. (Photo by Behrooz Modarai, reproduced from Lawton, M. P., Newcomer, R. J., and Byerts, T. O. _Community Planning for an Aging Society_, with permission of Dowden, Hutchinson, and Ross, publishers.)

(Lawton, 1970b). However, organizational assistance by administration or a floor tenant group can encourage their use by small groups. In good climates a common outdoor balcony can also serve the same purpose. The same study showed that a single-loaded corridor with outdoor exposure was heavily used for sitting in good weather and was associated with a much higher level of social interaction than in another part of the same building where the traditional double-loaded corridor design was used (Lawton, 1970b).

The need for privacy exists in all of us; the need is often frustrated in older people living with other family members. In planned housing, it is standard to provide private living units that are not shared with unrelated individuals (except in unusual instances, by request), with private bathrooms. Cost considerations have led to the 'efficiency' unit (combined living room and bedroom) as the norm. However, where possible a separate bedroom and some way to shut off the kitchen from the living area are desirable. For those who do not like to be observed as they walk through the lobby, an alternative entrance to the elevators or living areas may make them more comfortable.

A number of planning decisions are required for new housing. Site choice is subject to many of the same considerations discussed under 'neighbourhood' above. One of the earliest decisions to be made is whether to build for older people only or whether to house people of widely varying ages. Social science research in the USA has been quite clear in demonstrating that there are advantages associated with age-segregated housing, including a higher level of social interaction (Rosow, 1967) and a variety of other indicators of well-being (Teaff, Lawton, Nahemow, and Carlson, 1973). While part of the advantage is due to the greater personal security in high crime areas, there are other good reasons mentioned above why social integration may be easier among age peers. On the other hand, surveys of urban aged suggest that only about one-third would actively choose age-segregated housing if they were to move (Lawton, 1976a). This suggests that while many people's needs may best be met in an age-dense environment, the majority with housing needs would be deprived if age-integrated living were not available. The task of governmental policy makers is thus seen to be the encouragement of new housing environments where ages are integrated while at the same time ensuring that the critical mass of elderly is adequate to allow the choice of age peers when desired. It is also important that the age mix not include vulnerable elderly and problem children or teenagers, as is so frequent in the public housing programme of the USA. The age-integrated setting will have the best chance for success if accompanied by a strong administrative commitment to the idea of inter-generational living and the provision of both age-specific and controlled interactive spaces and programmes. Thus, a children's playground may provide rewarding spectator and social participation opportunities for the elderly, but they should not be forced by spatial design to traverse this area except by choice.

Similarly, a senior activity area should be located and access to it controlled so that it is limited to older people. Other spaces where behaviour is easily monitored by staff or responsible tenants may be used for planned events by people of all ages.

Many assertions have been made about the desirability of planning small housing estates so as to encourage closer relationships among elderly tenants and between warden and tenants. Research done in 153 such estates in the USA, ranging from 10 to over 600 units, failed to show any relationship between size and tenant indicators such as housing satisfaction, social interaction, or participation in activities (Lawton, Nahemow, and Teaff, 1975). Thus, where the

economics of the situation demand larger estates, there seem
to be no disadvantages from tenants' point of view.

There has also been a similar negative feeling toward
high rise structures. The Lawton et al study did find that
tenants living in low rise structures or in lower floors of
high rise structures were more satisfied with their housing
and were more mobile in the outside community than were
residents of high rise structures or those living in upper
floors. Thus, where there is a choice, lower structures
are preferable. Where land scarcity requires a high rise
building, the staff must be alerted to take counteractive
measures, such as providing incentives for interaction with
the local community or allowing dissatisfied residents of
upper floors to move into vacant lower floor flats.

Another planning decision with major spatial implications involves the kinds of services to be provided in
addition to basic shelter. While all such housing should
have informal and formal activity space, there is much controversy over whether other services such as communal meals,
medical services, personal care, or housekeeping help should
be provided. Elderly tenants' own preferences are very
strong for having some form of on-site medical care available
(Lawton, 1969; Carp, 1976). An unobtrusive form, such as a
physician's office is preferred over the more explicitly
illness-connoting infirmary or nursing care section. Lawton
(1976b) found that supportive services were associated with
increased housing satisfaction, but also with a decreased
level of interaction with the outside community. These
findings suggest that many of these services may be best
reserved for elderly tenants whose capabilities are mildly
impaired but who are not ready for an institution. For the
normally independent, the necessity for doing one's own
shopping, cooking, and housecleaning, and seeking medical
care in the community exercises and maintains their capabilities. However, even if a housing environment begins operation with highly capable tenants, long range planning must
either include provision for future service-delivery space
or face the unsavoury task of transferring tenants elsewhere
as their competence becomes marginal.

In any case, for either initial construction or later
remodelling, the common dining space will be a major social
centre and special care should be taken to create a warm,
aesthetically pleasing atmosphere. Waitress rather than
cafeteria service reduces the institutional quality. Some
choice of two-, four- and possibly six-person tables should
be included to suit individual need. Total space requirements should be calculated to include the wider pathways

required by people in wheelchairs or walkers. Since people
tend to gather near the dining room about half an hour before
service, and many will remain after the meal, a comfortable
lounge or gallery with seating will enhance the social quality of the occasion. Space for a medical clinic should be
designed to look as much like a community physician's office
as possible, with a waiting room. The decor should de-
emphasize the 'sick' atmosphere since research suggests that
it is very anxiety-arousing for the well elderly to be
reminded of sickness (Greenbaum, Lawton and Singer, 1970).
If the housing includes an infirmary or nursing care section,
these should be zoned so as to allow access to the independent
tenant areas but not have pathways that require the independent to observe the more frankly medical-care sections. It
is particularly desirable to have medical dispensary care
for the independent located away from the more institutional
areas.

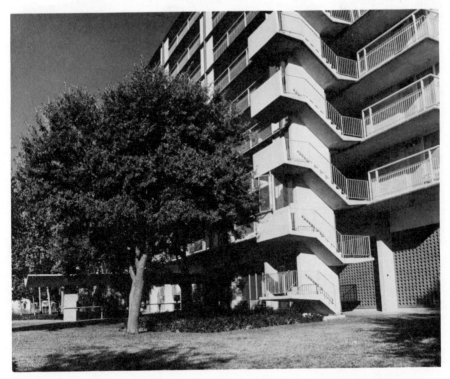

Figure 7:   Low cost public housing can be aesthetically
pleasing. The contemporary style of Victoria Plaza, San
Antonio, Texas, is much appreciated by its elderly tenants.
(Photo by Collas Smelzer, Thomas Thompson, architect.)

Finally, care should be taken to see that the finish materials, decor, and style of the housing do not in themselves convey society's negative stereotypes about aging. Bare concrete, cinder-block walls, uncarpeted floors, stark exteriors, and obviously cheap materials connote second class citizenship. Unusual architectural lines, a beautiful overhang, balconies, non-institutional furniture, indoor or outdoor plantings promote a sense of pride that adds significantly to the self-concept of the older tenant.

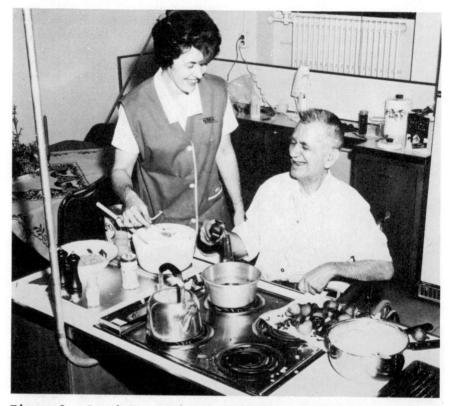

Figure 8: Specially designed dwelling-unit features increase the perceived competence of handicapped people. (Photo courtesy of Administration on Aging, United States Department of Health, Education, and Welfare.)

Community-based dwelling-unit design

Most household units were built with the average adult user in mind and with relatively little concern for livability in general. Many of the design considerations that are

therapeutic for the elderly represent good design for people
in general and may be incorporated in new construction.
Many millions of older people live in older units that are
unsafe, unaesthetic, or competence-reducing, however. A
major task for the future involves the development of a
financial base for remodelling or reconstruction and the
design expertise to guide such rehabilitation of existing
units, neither of which now exists. In particular, it should
be possible to develop sets of guidelines for the minimizing
of barriers and hazards, the rearrangement of furniture,
first aid minor remodelling, and major remodelling that could
be used by sub-professional household design service workers
to help elderly occupants make their homes more livable.

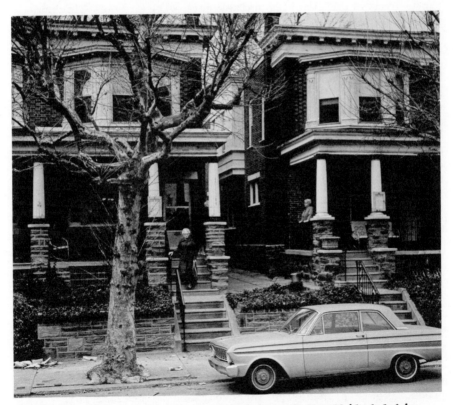

Figure 9:   Older homes in the vicinity of the Philadelphia
Geriatric Center were inexpensively remodelled to provide
independent living for three older people each. (Photo by
Lindelle Studio. Reproduced from Lawton, M.P., Newcomer,
R.J., and Byerts, T.O., Community Planning for an Aging
Society, with permission of Dowden, Hutchinson, and Ross,
publishers.)

A number of attempts to make better use of existing housing
are now in progress on a demonstration basis. In Kansas
City an attempt was made to interest older people in the
cooperative sharing of large houses with a live-in warden,
but few people who wished to live this way could be located
(Peterson and Sigler, 1976). The public housing authority
of Plainfield, New Jersey, is in the process of brokering
the conversion of homes owned by older people into two separate units, with the additional created unit offering income
to the owner and a private apartment for an elderly renter.
The Philadelphia Geriatric Center bought inexpensive houses
near the parent institution and made single bedrooms available to elderly renters. The necessity for sharing kitchen
and bathroom caused inter-personal problems and this model
was abandoned. Its present 'community housing' model created
three individual dwelling units, each with private kitchen,
bathroom, and bed-sitting room. The three units share only
the front entrance and front parlour/television room. Research has shown this model to be eminently successful (Brody,
Kleban and Lawton, 1975; Kleban and Turner-Massey, 1976).
Liebowitz (1976) has reviewed a number of other alternative
housing modes that have been attempted in the USA, though
none other than the Philadelphia Geriatric Center's has been
subjected to research evaluation. There are obvious difficulties involved when relatively independent older people
are forced to share living spaces. It may well be that true
communal arrangements will work best for people of limited
competence who live under some supervised arrangement. It
is likely that future generations of older people will be
even less tolerant of limitations on their privacy.

Another form of household sharing is the situation where
an older person lives with a relative. In 1970 about 20 per
cent of the older people in the USA lived with a relative,
less than nine per cent with an adult child. The latter
figure represents a nearly 50 per cent reduction since 1940.
The evidence seems clear that increased industrialization of
a country reduces the number of such shared households and
that older people themselves increasingly wish to maintain
households independent of younger family members as their
economic capability improves (Shanas et al, 1969). In the
face of such a large scale social change, it does not seem
productive to plan design interventions to reverse this
trend, for the majority of relatively healthy older people..
On the other hand, there does appear to be some basis for
social and physical programming that would make it easier
for a younger family to share its household with an older
person of limited competence, in the hope of prolonging
community residence and avoiding institutionalization. Life
in such households is often stressful for both generations,

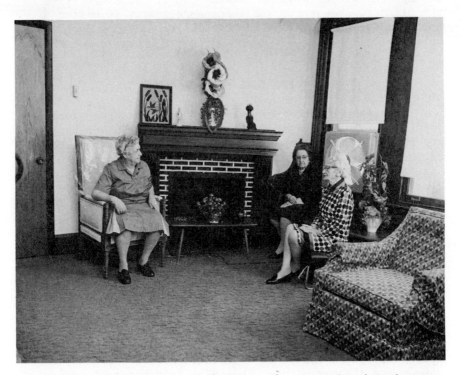

Figure 10: The original living room is the only shared space for the three residents of the remodelled homes. Each resident has a complete private living unit. (Photo by Lindelle Studios.)

often revolving about such issues as privacy, isolation, the sharing of kitchen and bathroom, and the loss of or maintenance of roles such as cooking and housekeeping. There is much to be said for a dwelling-unit design now available in some countries (Japan, Spain) that permits the household to be zoned so as to produce private space for both generations (bedroom, toilet, cooking facilities, dwelling-unit entrance) as well as shared space. A choice is thus available for private or shared activity as desired. Where the older person's deficit is great enough to require surveillance, household engineering could also be done to reduce hazards, such as limiting egress from a 'safe' area, disconnecting an existing stove, and so on.

Clearly, guidelines regarding the design and redesign of 'normal' dwelling-units are sparse, and research knowledge almost nonexistent. Nonetheless, it is felt that knowledge of the typical deficits associated with old age, and of

neighbourhoods and planned housing can at least sensitize
the planner, architect, and service-deliverer in making
specific design decisions in relation to existing dwelling-
units.

INSTITUTIONS FOR THE AGED

Despite the fact that only five per cent of the elderly
population in the USA is institutionalized, a disproportionate amount of attention has been devoted to this population
in both the gerontological and the environmental design
literature. Reasons for this overemphasis are obvious. The
cost of such care is tremendous, and the institution is thus
the focus of a major problem for the entire society. The
quality of life in many institutions is deplorable and the
need for improvement has stimulated workers disproportionately. Finally, institutionalized people are on 'display'
literally 24 hours per day and thus are far easier to use
as subjects by research workers.

The major problem involved in defining desirable and
undesirable physical characteristics of institutions by
social scientific research is the absence of usable criteria
for good and bad institutions. Most people who enter institutions die there (or in an associated hospital); thus, one
cannot use discharge rate, length of institutionalization,
or post-discharge community tenure as criteria against which
to validate institutional variations. The great bulk of
the environmental literature in this area thus accepts the
a priori judgment that such attributes as aesthetic quality,
provision of privacy, opportunity for social interaction,
the delivery of medical and social services, and the achieve-
ment of meaningful time use represent desirable institutional qualities.

Most institutions have an essential health care component. Too often this component dominates the entire milieu
so as to preclude the possibility of achieving a sense of
warmth and concern for needs other than physical health and
security. These are of course, bare minimum requirements
for an institution; but most building standards concern only
physical safety and do not consider ways in which livability
may be affected by rigid life-safety standards. Institutions
as a class demand conformity, standardized practices, loss
of individual initiative, and a wall of separation between
the institution and the community. Thus one has long hallways, shared facilities, scheduled times for almost every
behaviour, a loss of privacy, proscription of most personal
possessions, staff work to substitute for residents' self-

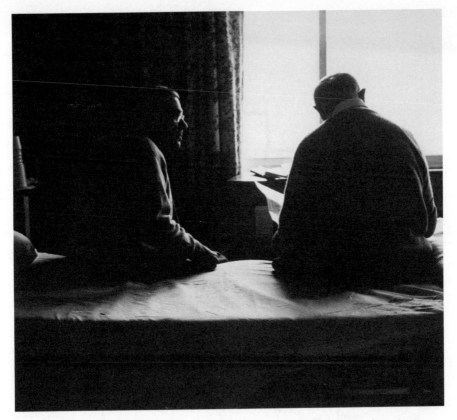

Figure 11: Hospital beds for those who do not require bed care are both difficult to sit on and contribute to an institutional atmosphere. (Photo courtesy of Administration on Aging, United States Department of Health, Education and Welfare.)

maintaining behaviour, and physical uniformity, all in the name either of the need for health care or the maintenance of a mass organization. Necessary as some of these features are, the application of human behaviour principles to institutional design may radically improve the quality of life for elderly residents.

The Philadelphia Geriatric Center has recently completed a building designed with these principles clearly in mind. Since this represented such as unusual opportunity to incorporate existing knowledge and theory into institutional design, an extended description of its innovative design features will be presented here, followed by a consideration of other aspects of design that were not utilized in this building.

260

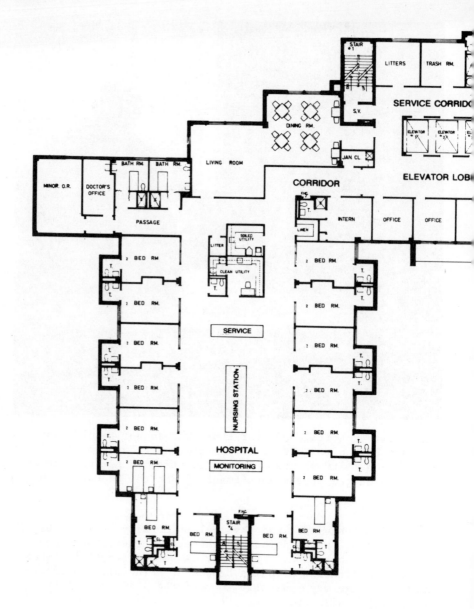

Figure 12: The Weiss Institute of the Philadelphia Geriatric
Center (wing on right) was designed with the needs of the
mentally impaired aged in mind. (Demchik, Berger, and Dash,
architects.)

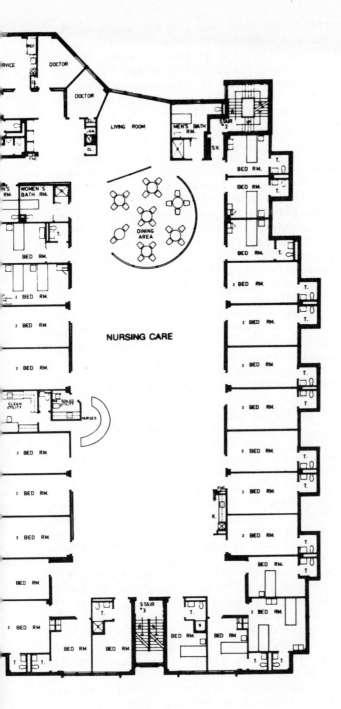

The Weiss Institute was designed for the needs of the older person with massive behavioural deficits resulting from senile dementia and related conditions. About half of all people in long term care institutions suffer from some degree of mental impairment, which is evidenced by memory loss, intellectual loss, disorientation, deterioration of personal habits, and loss of social skills. The following design features were included:

a)   A very large (40' x 80') central space around which residents' bedrooms are ranged. This 'sociopetal' design (Osmond, 1957) was deemed especially helpful to the mentally impaired aged for several reasons. First, a far greater visual expanse is available to the resident from almost any vantage point; his orientation is enhanced because he can see all of the important areas from the entrance to his room or from any other point. Second, since the central area must be traversed in order to travel from one location to another, encounters between residents are facilitated, which is a necessary prior condition for social interaction. Third, the large space allows the scheduling of most activities in a location where at the very least something interesting to watch is provided, and at best, the non-participant may be motivated to participate by seeing others do so. Finally, the inevitable crowding of the typically long institutional hallway is totally dispensed with.

b)   The dining room is marked off from the central area by an attractive pole divider and is thus clearly a 'new' locale to which residents travel for meals, but it is visually accessible through the divider as a reminder of the next meal, an important aid in orientation to time.

c)   The centre space itself is articulated into components. First, an 8 foot 'corridor' is indicated around the periphery by a darker floor and a lowered ceiling, which provides some orientational cues as well as conforming to code requirements that there by an 8 foot 'corridor'. Second, the largest section is designated as an informal social space and articulated by furniture, whose location is changed for different purposes. Third, the 'centrepiece' (not shown in Figure 12, but placed in centre to the right of the nurses' station) is an aesthetically designed garden gazebo with seats and live plants inside; attached to and forming both a structural and an aesthetic component of the gazebo is an exercise rail and steps to be used in physical therapy. Fourth, the area beyond the gazebo is designed for scheduled activities, such as occupational therapy, discussion groups, slide shows, or music therapy, where some isolation from the larger area is desirable. Finally, a small kitchen that is used by residents

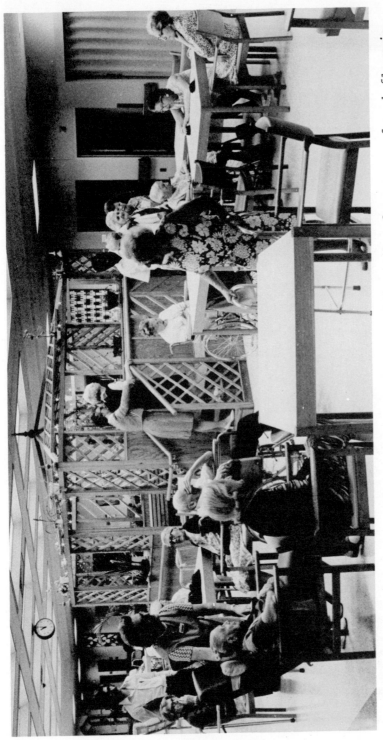

Figure 13: Centre of social life and therapy is large open space that forms core of each floor in Weiss Institute. Since residents' rooms cluster around this centre they are attracted to participate in activities. Residents, staff, visitors and volunteers all mingle here, with health stimulating effect.

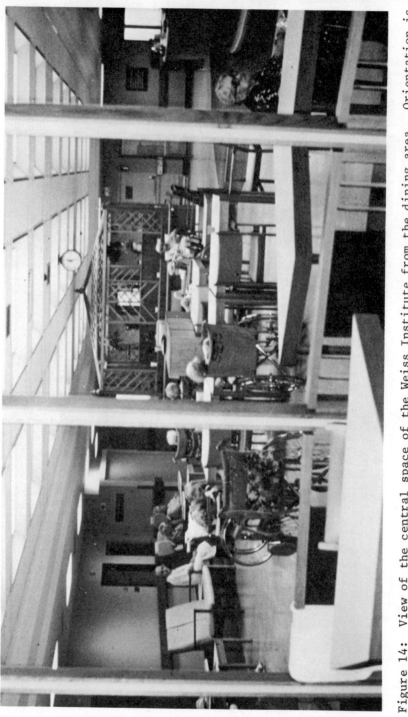

Figure 14: View of the central space of the Weiss Institute from the dining area. Orientation is aided by being able to see from almost any vantage point where eating takes place.

under supervision opens onto the centre space, but may be closed off at other times.

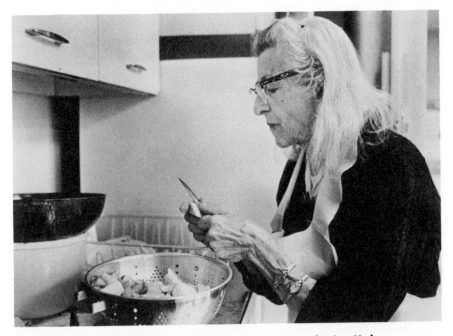

Figure 15: Pullman kitchen on each floor of the Weiss Institute is an important aid in arousing interest of those whose life was involved in preparing meals for their families.

d)   A lounge separate from the central space but with one side open to view is provided for TV and is heavily utilized by family visitors and residents.

e)   All rooms are two-person or single rooms with a separate toilet/washroom, allowing a greater degree of privacy than usually provided.

f)   The colours of each room are carefully varied so as to allow the occupant to differentiate his/her own room in terms of matching door frame, wall colour, and furnishing colour; the presence of four such colour ensembles allows the resident to distinguish her room from those of near neighbours. While there is at present no research data to suggest that one colour is any more 'therapeutic' than another, high contrast between colours, as well as bright and decisively-hued colours have been shown to have a favourable effect on the ability of the elderly to negotiate their environments (Pastalan et al, 1973).

g)   A variety of other orientational aids were used, such as:

- Different elevator-area colours for each floor, with large signs and maps indicating the locations of significant areas.

- Large-size three-dimensional room numbers outside each resident room, placed at average eye height.

- Large-lettered names of occupant(s) on room doors.

- 'Reality-orientation' boards, allowing staff to indicate the building name, floor, season, date and day of week, next meal, and weather.

h)   The furniture was carefully chosen. The 'Scandiform' chair was designed with attention to such matters as the height, width, depth, and slope requirements for elderly residents, and is adjustable in these dimensions. They also have removable wings for headrest and tables.

i)   Heavy and pleasantly smooth textured handrails were designed especially for the elderly.

j)   Many other features were included to improve the aesthetic quality of the institutional environment, such as plants (all known to be non-toxic if eaten), cheerful wall hangings, framed pictures, and a personal bulletin board for each resident.

k)   Illumination level was designed so as to provide daylight equivalent light in all areas whenever desired, with controls allowing selective reduction of this level when desired.

l)   Staff offices are proximate to resident areas. The nursing station is an open freestanding structure that allows residents access to nursing staff and an unimpeded view of the entire floor by staff at the station.

A research evaluation of the impact of this building will shortly be completed. It is important to note that the Weiss Institute concept would not be appropriate for some other elderly user groups. Institutional residents who are relatively capable, mentally and physically, would have their

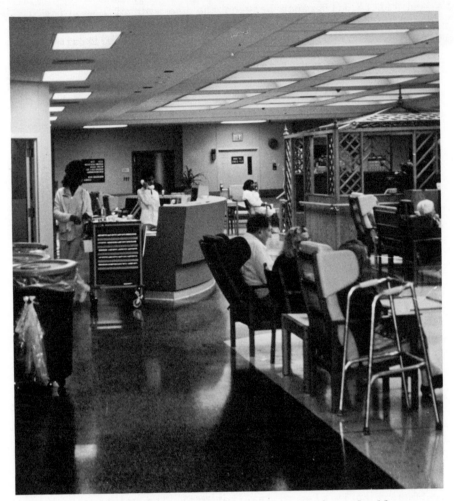

Figure 16: Not only do nurses have a full view of all areas of the unit, but they and the residents are encouraged to interact by the lack of a physical barrier between the nurses station and the resident area.

life space grossly constricted by the forced centring of most activity in the central area. While Weiss Institute residents do have a choice among private, small-social, and large-social space, they have no privacy at all for much of the day that they typically spend in the central section.

Some other more general therapeutic uses of physical design may be of interest. The neighbourhood location of an institution that serves the physically ill seems less critical than in the case of housing. For example, Lipman (1968)

found little difference between the use made of community
resources in homes for the aged located proximate to or
distant from local centres. Where there are few impairments
(as in board-and-care homes), the locational decisions applying to housing are more relevant.

As in the case of housing, there has been much debate
over the issue of institutional size as it relates to quality
of care. Research on this question has come up with conflicting results (Anderson et al, 1969; Gottesman, 1974); at
present most data suggest that factors other than size are
more important determinants of institutional quality.

The heterogeneity vs. homogeneity issue in the institution centres on the mixing of residents functioning at low
and high levels of mental competence. In practice, most
institutions segregate the brain-damaged and those with
severe behavioural problems from the more competent. For
the Weiss Institute study, people with a somewhat broader
range of impairment (though still within the impaired range)
were mixed and our consumer survey of both staff and relatives revealed a strong conviction that this relative heterogeneity was destructive to the better off residents; unfortunately, the high level of impairment among residents
precluded a similar survey of their attitudes. The mix was
readjusted to the more usual segregation by mental competence
situation. Although to date there is no hard direct evidence
to document whether there is either a destructive effect on
the competent or a behaviour-elevating effect on the less
competent, the indirect evidence would seem to favour zoning
institutional areas so as not to mix pathways and to avoid
visual access between the relatively well and the deteriorated.

Many of the same considerations regarding social spaces
in housing apply also to institutions. The relative lack
of locomotion ability in nursing home residents makes even
more desirable the location of such spaces where there is a
high density of pedestrian traffic. Staff and visitors will
frequently object to the sight of residents appearing to sit
totally inactive, especially immediately inside or outside
a main entrance where they present a 'bad face to the community'. The designer should be firm in insisting to the spon-
soring group that this negative quality is more than compen-
sated for in the enrichment provided for those who enjoy
watching or finding companionship in such a location. Similarly, there has been a marked tendency to locate social
spaces at the ends of corridors. While there are some who
enjoy such a quiet retreat, this should not substitute for
a relatively large informal space near the entrance to the
area or the nurses station, the two usual centres of activity.

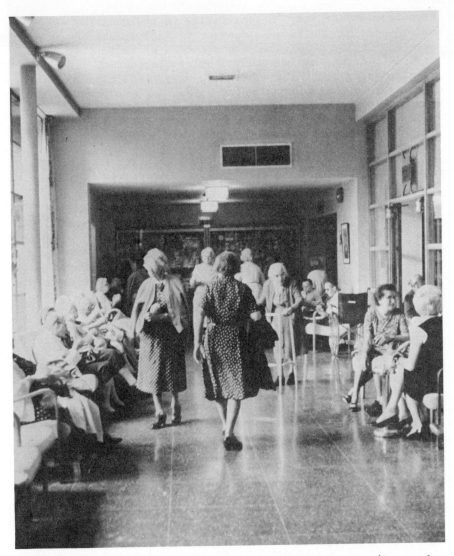

Figure 17: The main lobby of an institution is heavily used for both social interaction and more passive, but enjoyable, watching of activity. (Photo by Jeanne Bader.)

Such a room should have a substantial opening with a full view of these centres for most occupants of the space.

Institutions are notorious for their active particip-ation in allowing residents' remaining skills to atrophy. While much of this problem is on the human level (i.e. staff's finding it more efficient to do a task for the resident rather than allowing her to do it, however faltering, for herself), the designer's sensitivity to the need for skill maintenance may persuade a sponsor to include the physical necessities for doing so. The presence of facilities for washing, drying, and possibly ironing clothes may serve as a reminder to staff that there can be satisfaction for some residents in these instrumental tasks. An open small kitchen for more competent residents, and one that can be used as part of a supervised activity programme for more impaired people not only maintains skill but may stimulate positive affective experiences associated with eating and sharing food with others. Instrumental tasks suitable for men of today's generation of elderly are more difficult to devise. A sheltered workshop might be considered, since many of these tasks are consonant with the masculine self-concept and are perceived as 'productive'. Spaces for planned activities, crafts and hobbies for the fully mobile resident need not be located near high traffic areas, since these users will be willing to walk to them. However, adequate service cannot be given to the more restricted unless storage and work space is available on the residential floor. The Weiss Institute, rather than committing permanent space for such built-in furniture, uses storage cabinets and working surfaces that may be rolled to any desired location within the large central space.

The nostalgic view is often expressed that warmth can be conveyed only through 'traditional' decor, which is presumed to be liked better by the elderly because it is more familiar. Some small institutions have, in fact, most successfully created a warm atmosphere by assembling non-institutional furniture as if in a private home. While there is no relevant information on this issue, in practice it has seemed that institutional residents respond positively, as do people in general, to furniture and materials that are attractive and that connote a caring intent, rather than responding to one particular style or the other. The trouble with the usual 'institutional' or 'decorator' atmosphere lies in the failure of the designer or sponsor to care enough to consider the psychological and social needs of the user in furnishing an institution, even if it costs somewhat more, rather than in the use of 'modern' styles per se.

There are necessarily many omissions in this brief resume. Fortunately, an excellent, highly design-specific sourcebook is available and is mandatory for those seeking to upgrade the quality of the institutional environment (Koncelik, 1976).

CONCLUSION

The major point of this presentation is that the quality of life for elderly target groups may be improved significantly through environmental design. In order to accomplish this goal the first requirement is awareness of the facts about aging and sensitivity to the special needs of this group. Beyond this point, some empirical research is available as a further guide, and there is every reason to think that more will shortly be forthcoming. The successful application of such knowledge depends, of course, on the collaborative effects of the designer, the sponsor and administrative personnel, and someone with expertise in aging, whether a gerontological generalist or a specialist in the environmental psychology of later life. Interchange among such people is not always easy: the designer may feel defensive about criticism in his specialty, the sponsor is necessarily concerned over cost, the gerontologist may be unrealistic in his demands or arrogant when taking the role of the designer, and so on. However, these are necessary costs incurred in developing a good product. Finally, it may be noted that the older person herself as a source of design-relevant input has not been mentioned in the discussion. No process of planning should occur without a significant effort by all members of a planning team to seek such input, by talking with articulate elderly informants, tenant councils, senior citizen groups, or even doing formal pre-planning surveys. While some consumer studies of older people's preferences have appeared in the literature (e.g. Carp, 1976), the real-life flavour of older people's needs can never be experienced without direct contact.

REFERENCES

ANDERSON, N. N., HOLMBERG, R. H., SCHNEIDER, R. E., and
STONE, L. A. (1969) Policy issues regarding nursing
homes, American Rehabilitation Foundation, Minneapolis.

ASHFORD, N., and HOLLOWAY, F. M. (1972) "Transportation
patterns of older people in six urban centers",
Gerontologist, 12, pp.43-47.

BALTES, P. B., and LABOUVIE, G. V. (1973) "Adult development
of intellectual performance: description, explanation,
and modification", in C. Eisdorfer and M. P. Lawton
(eds.) The psychology of adult development and aging,
American Psychological Association, Washington.

BENNETT, R., and ECKMAN, J. (1973) "Attitudes toward aging",
in C. Eisdorfer and M. P. Lawton (eds.) The psychology
of adult development and aging, American Psychological
Association, Washington.

BEYER, G., and WOODS, M. E. (1963) Living and activity
patterns of the aged, Cornell University Center for
Housing and Environmental Studies, Ithaca, New York.

BRODY, E., KLEBAN, M., and LAWTON, M. P. (1975) "Intermediate
housing for the elderly", Gerontologist, 15, pp.350-356.

BROTMAN, H. B. (1976) "Every tenth American - the 'problem'
of aging", in M. P. Lawton, R. J. Newcomer, and
T. O. Byerts (eds.) Community planning for an aging
society, Dowden, Hutchinson, and Ross, Stroudsburg, PA.

BUTLER, R. N. (1969) "Age-ism: another form of bigotry",
Gerontologist, 9, pp.243-246.

BUTLER, R. N. (1975) Why survive?, Harper and Row, New York.

BUTLER, R. N., and LEWIS, M. I. (1973) Aging and mental
health, Mosby, St. Louis.

BYERTS, T. O. (ed.) (1973) Housing and environment for the elderly, Gerontological Society, Washington.

BYERTS, T. O. (1976) "Reflecting user requirements in designing city parks", in M. P. Lawton, R. J. Newcomer, and T. O. Byerts, Community planning for an aging society, Dowden, Hutchinson, and Ross, Stroudsburg, PA.

CARP, F. M. (1966) A future for the aged, University of Texas Press, Austin.

CARP, F. M. (1971) "Public transit and retired people", in E. J. Cantilli and J. L. Schmelzer (eds.) Transportation and aging: selected issues, Administration on Aging, Washington, DC.

CARP, F. M. (1976) "User evaluation of housing for the elderly", Gerontologist, 16, pp.102–111.

CUMMING, E., and HENRY, W. E. (1961) Growing old, Basic Books, New York.

FISKE, D. W., and MADDI, S. R. (eds.) (1961) Functions of varied experience, Dorsey, Homewood, IL.

GOLANT, S. M. (1976) "Intraurban transportation needs and problems of the elderly", in M. P. Lawton, R. J. Newcomer, and T. O. Byerts (eds.) Community planning for an aged society, Dowden, Hutchinson, and Ross, Stroudsburg, PA.

GOTTESMAN, L. E. (1974) "Nursing home performance as related to resident traits, ownership, size, and source of payments", American Journal of Public Health, 64, pp.269–276.

GREEN, I., FEDEWA, B. E., JOHNSTON, C. A., JACKSON, W. M., and DEERDORFF, H. L. (1975) Housing for the elderly: the development and design process, Van Nostrand, New York.

GREENBAUM, M. B., LAWTON, M. P., and SINGER, M. (1970)
"Tenant perceptions of health, health services, and
status in two apartment buildings for the elderly",
Aging and Human Development, 1, pp.333-344.

KLEBAN, M., and TURNER-MASSEY, P. (1976) "The impact of
intermediate housing on tenants and their domains of
well-being compared with control groups", paper presented
for annual meeting, Gerontological Society, New York,
October.

KONCELIK, J. (1976) Designing the open nursing home, Dowden,
Hutchinson, and Ross, Stroudsburg, PA.

LAWTON, M. P. (1969) "Supportive services in the context of
the housing environment", Gerontologist, 9, pp.15-19.

LAWTON, M. P. (1970a) "Ecology and aging", in L. Pastalan
and D. H. Carson (eds.) The spatial behaviour of older
people, University of Michigan, Institute of Gerontology,
Ann Arbor.

LAWTON, M. P. (1970b) "Public behaviour of older people in
congregate housing", in J. Archea and C. Eastman (eds.)
Environmental Design Research Association II, pp.372-380,
Carnegie-Mellon University, Pittsburgh.

LAWTON, M. P. (1975) Planning and managing housing for the
elderly, Wiley-Interscience, New York.

LAWTON, M. P. (1976a) "Homogeneity and heterogeneity in
housing for the elderly", in M. P. Lawton, R. J. Newcomer
and T. O. Byerts (eds.) Community planning for an aging
society, Dowden, Hutchinson, and Ross, Stroudsburg, PA.

LAWTON, M. P. (1976b) "The relative impact of congregate
and traditional housing on elderly tenants", Gerontologist,
16, pp.237-242.

LAWTON, M. P. (in press) "Social science methods for
evaluating the quality of housing for the elderly",
Journal of Architectural Research.

LAWTON, M. P. and COHEN, J. (1974) "The generality of
housing impact on the well-being of older people",
Journal of Gerontology, 29, pp.194-204.

LAWTON, M. P., NAHEMOW, L., and TEAFF, J. (1975) "Housing
characteristics and the well-being of elderly tenants
in federally-assisted housing", Journal of Gerontology,
30, pp.601-607.

LAWTON, M. P., NAHEMOW, L., YAFFE, S. and FELDMAN, S. (1976)
"Psychological impact of crime and fear of crime: the
elderly and public housing", in J. Goldsmith and
S. Goldsmith (eds.) Crime and the elderly: challenge
and response, Heath, New York.

LAWTON, M. P., NEWCOMER, R. J., and BYERTS, T. O. (eds.)
(1976) Community planning for an aging society,
Dowden, Hutchinson, and Ross, Stroudsburg, PA.

LIEBOWITZ, B. (1976) "Implications of the project for
policy and planning", paper presented at annual meeting
of Gerontological Society, New York. October.

LIPMAN, A. (1968) "A socio-architectural view of life in
three homes for old people", Gerontologia Clinica, 10,
pp.88-101.

LOWENTHAL, M. F. and BOLER, D. (1965) "Voluntary vs.
involuntary social withdrawal", Journal of Gerontology,
20, pp.363-371.

NATIONAL CENTER FOR HEALTH STATISTICS (1967) Prevalence of
chronic conditions and impairments among residents of
housing and personal care homes, USPHS Publication
No. 1000, Series 12, No. 8, US Government Printing
Office, Washington, DC.

NEWCOMER, R. J. (1973) "Housing, services, and neighborhood activities", paper presented at annual meeting of the Gerontological Society, Miami Beach.

OSMOND, H. (1957) "Function as the basis of psychiatric ward design", Mental Hospitals, 8, pp.23-30.

PASTALAN, L. A., MAUTZ, R. K., and MERRIL, J. (1973) "The simulation of age-related losses", in W. F. E. Preiser (ed.) Environmental Design Research, Vol.1, Dowden, Hutchinson, and Ross, Stroudsburg, PA.

PERIN, C. (1970) With man in mind, MIT Press, Cambridge, MA.

PETERSON, W., and SIGLER, J. (1976) Alternative living arrangements: an attempt to use existing housing for group living among the elderly, Institute for Community Studies, Kansas City, MO.

RILEY, M. W. and FONER, A. (1968) Aging and society, Vol.1, Russell Sage Foundation, New York.

ROSOW, I. (1967) Social integration of the aged, Free Press, New York.

SHANAS, E., TOWNSEND, P., WEDDERBURN, D., FRIIS, H., MILHOJ, P., and STEHOUWER, J. (1968) Old people in three industrial societies, Atherton, New York.

SHERWOOD, S., GRIER, D. S., MORRIS, J. N., and SHERWOOD, C. C. (1972) The Highland Heights Experiment, US Department of Housing and Urban Development, Washington, DC.

TEAFF, J., LAWTON, M. P., NAHEMOW, L., and CARLSON, D. (1978) "Impact of age integration on the well-being of elderly tenants in public housing", Journal of Gerontology, 33, pp.126-133.

US DEPARTMENT OF HEALTH, EDUCATION, AND WELFARE (1973) New facts about older Americans, DHEW Publication No.(SRS) 73-20006, US Government Printing Office, Washington, DC.

Homes for Old People:
Towards a Positive Environment

ALAN LIPMAN AND ROBERT SLATER

INTRODUCTION

In this paper[1] the case is presented for a set of design
proposals for local authority Homes for old people. The
discussion is in three parts. The first highlights a key
consideration in the operational philosophy underlying the
proposals - the goal of minimizing residents' dependence on
staff. This discussion pinpoints certain features of institutional accommodation for old people held to counter
the positive basis of the goal. The second part deals with
what have been taken as the problematic social and organizational issues on which realization of the goal rests.
These are: encouraging personal and group activities among
residents, providing for resident privacy, and integrating
various categories of residents (principally 'confused' and
'rational' residents and those who are physically disabled
and able). The final section describes how these issues
and the related goal of independence have influenced the
design proposals.

THE OPERATIONAL PHILOSOPHY

The arguments in this paper are based on a particular
'operational philosophy'. That is, the proposals described
below stem from a specific value orientation. They illustrate the application, in this instance, to residential
Homes, of a principle which we believe ought to govern
provision of services for elderly people who are deemed to
require 'care and attention'. For a summary description of
these services see the Personal Social Services Council's
interim report (1975).

In an analogous context - designing for young mentally
handicapped people - Gunzburg and Gunzburg (1973) have opted
for a rehabilitative philosophy. They stressed the therapeutic potentialities of selected physical elements and
spatial arrangements. These they sought to direct toward
raising mentally handicapped people's "levels of functioning"
to enable them to live in "the open community". A therapeutic perspective of this nature has, however, limited
relevance to people in the concluding stage of their life
cycles. In particular, it seems inappropriate for those
aged whose straitened personal and social circumstances in
'open' communities constitute the very grounds on which
social service agencies define them as being in need of
residential care (e.g. Townsend, 1962; Tunstall, 1966; and
Meacher, 1972). For them a more apt perspective is one
that recognizes, perhaps reluctantly, the implications of
terminal residence exemplified by Townsend's depiction of
Homes as "last refuges". Such recognition implies, we contend, a philosophy orientated to maintaining residents'
independence and which, in operation, seeks to exploit the
potentialities of the physical environment.

Like Lindsley's (1964), our approach is prosthetic.
It assumes relatively unalterable disabilities, those accom-
panying aging (Kastenbaum, 1965), and seeks environmental
supports that can help maintain personal and social levels
of functioning. Granting man's present inability effectively to retard human aging processes, Lindsley advocated
attempts to compensate by means of physical aids for the
"behavioral debilitations" elderly people experience, as
have others (e.g. Lawton, 1970 and 1974). As indicated
below, our approach is to counter certain of the debilit-
ative and negative effects of institutional life noted by
Goffman (1961) and, dealing directly with accommodation for
the elderly, by Bennett and Nahemow (1965) and Meacher
(1972). Beyond this, by providing the relevant environmental amenities, it seeks to foster activities that appear
to fall within the capabilities of residents and so help
maintain their day-to-day levels of functioning.

Resident Independency and Institutional Life

Consider now the central tenet of the philosophy;
namely, minimizing residents' dependence on staff. Here
the nebulous notion of independence has been interpreted as
meaning "not contingent on...the action of others" (Onions,
1972). It has been viewed as an ideal state in which residents are not bound or subject to staff for conducting the

four broad categories of customary activity we have observed
in some thirty-seven Homes: the clusters of daily activities
that surround sleeping, toileting and bathing, preparing
and eating food, and socializing. The implications of this
ideal can probably best be conveyed by contrasting it with
the notion of hotel-like service embodied in the National
Assistance Act 1948, in terms of which local authority Homes
have been built since that date. Then, in seeking to abolish
workhouses the legislators envisaged substituting small
Homes modelled on residential hotels:

"The workhouse is doomed. Instead, local authorities
are busy planning and opening small, comfortable Homes, where
old people, many of them lonely, can live pleasantly and
with dignity. The old 'master and inmate' relationship is
being replaced by one more nearly approaching that of an
hotel manager and his guests" (Ministry of Health, 1950).

From this viewpoint, 'dignity' appears to reside in
being a guest for whom day-to-day services, often of an
intimate nature, are provided by others - a fostering of
dependence.

We believe the hotel model to be inappropriate. Even
if Homes functioned in this manner, and the evidence suggests
overwhelmingly that they do not (e.g. Townsend, 1962, and
Meacher, 1972), in our view dependency is inherent in the
notion. In particular, it militates against the independence
implicit in the voluntary, the contractual guest/manager
relationships suggested by the hotel model. It ignores the
asymmetric distribution of power in prevailing staff/resident
relationships. In addition, by proposing a reliance on
hotel-like personnel, the notion tends to entrench dependency. It subverts the expression of such potential for
self-help and mutual assistance as might exist among residents. Our design proposals seek to exploit such potentialities. Rather than viewing residents as passive recipients
of daily services, we have assumed that, with the aid of
supportive physical settings, they can be induced to exercise
the self-maintenance skills acquired throughout their lives.

Attempts to implement this stance give rise to congregate living conditions. They call for forms of grouped
accommodation, if only in consequence of the anticipated
mutual help furnished by fellow residents. And this is
reinforced by the necessity, we contend, for maintaining at
least the present standards of care afforded to residents
by 'domestic' and 'care attendant' staff. Here we are in a
dilemma. Both these circumstances of group living and the

presence of staff, are conducive to the dependent situations
we have noted (e.g. Slater, 1968, and Lipman, 1970) and
which have been attributed to the qualities of 'total instit-
utionality' of Homes by, for example, Bennett and Nahemow
(1965) and Snyder (1973). A preferred resolution of the
dilemma probably lies in applying the principle of maintaining the independence of 'at risk' elderly people before
they qualify for admittance to Homes. This calls for social
policies that obviate the grounds for institutional care.
Action of this nature has been urged, usually in the form
of domiciliary services (e.g. Townsend, 1962, and Committee
on Local Authority and Allied Personal Services, 1968). To
date, however, such services as exist have left the demand
for residential care unabated (Age Concern, 1973, and
Townsend, 1975). The quandary remains. At best, and this
is the purpose of our proposals, efforts can be made to
remove some of the factors that facilitate institutional
dependency.

Given this official emphasis in social policy, and the
Personal Social Services Council's (1975) forecast of its
persistence, our attention has, perforce, focused on the
Homes. Further, given the Council's similar expectation of
a continued shortage of trained staff (pp.27-30), our efforts
have tended to centre on physical design. In this context,
we have sought to draw on residents' resources; to enhance
their opportunities for self-sufficiency and minimize staff
intervention. With our prosthetic intentions in mind and
on the basis, principally, of our participant observation
studies (Harris, Lipman and Slater, 1977), attention has
been directed to the following areas of accommodation:

1.   The current provision of so-called bedsitting rooms
      (either for individual or multiple occupancy) that
      are insufficiently large to be used as such and whose
      layouts (e.g. positions of doors, windows and built-in
      fittings) prohibit a variety of furniture arrange-
      ments.

2.   Toilet and bathroom accommodation arranged in central-
      ized blocks (i.e. communally).

3.   Centralized dining rooms, and food preparation areas
      to which access is not customarily available to
      residents.

4.   Lengthy internal corridors.

5.   Access - doors opening directly into bedrooms (e.g.
      unscreened personal accommodation).

Figure 1 shows each of these points on a ground floor plan of one of the Homes we studied.

SOCIAL AND ORGANIZATIONAL ISSUES

In addition to this commitment to resident independency, our research experiences have led to three other related value orientations. Expressed, as they are, as articles of faith, these comprise the beliefs:

a) that activity, social and physical, on the part of the residents is likely to be more beneficial for them than the types of inactivity we have observed (e.g. Lipman, 1968) and which other investigators have reported (e.g. Anderson, 1963, and Meacher, 1972);

b) that privacy is a right, and that opportunities for personal and social privacy - for being alone or with chosen others - are, if exercised, likely to be beneficial (e.g. Pastalan, 1970, and Schwartz, 1975); and

c) that 'integrating' physically able and rational with frail and confused residents is likely to be advantageous for all - benefits for able and rational residents lie in the opportunity to accept responsibility for the care of their frail and confused fellow residents and for the latter in the assistance and stimulation afforded by the presence of the former (Meacher, 1972).

Activity

Our proposals are intended to provide physical settings in which residents' resources can be mobilized to counter symptoms of what Barton (1966) described as institutional neurosis, "a disease characterized by apathy, lack of initiative, loss of interest, especially in things of an impersonal nature, submissiveness...". Following Maslow's (1943) thesis on human motivation, among such resources we stress what he termed self-actualizing motives; acting in accord with desires, 'needs', to give expression to, to fulfil one's capabilities. In short, the proposals are intended to help foster, or reinforce, residents' abilities to 'do-things-for-themselves'. hopefully by minimizing the necessity for staff assistance - even for such an apparently trivial act as making oneself a cup of tea.

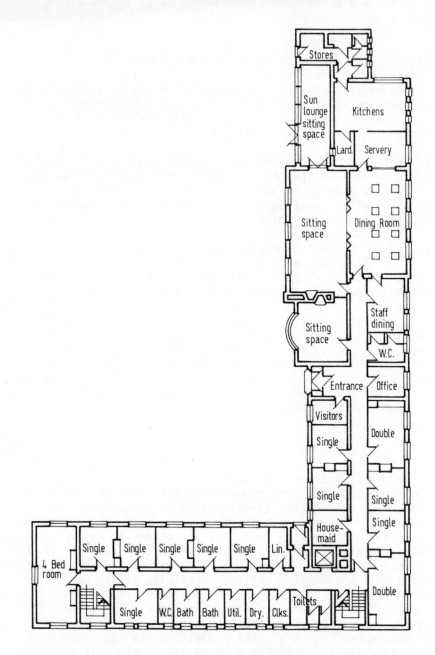

Figure 1: A typical plan of accommodation for old people

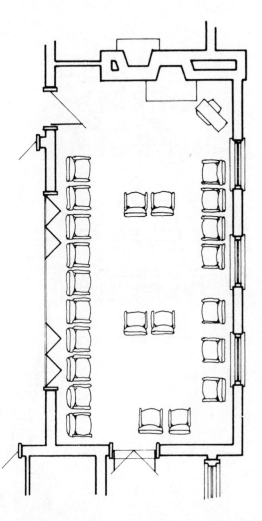

Figure 2: A conventional sitting room for twenty-three people

284

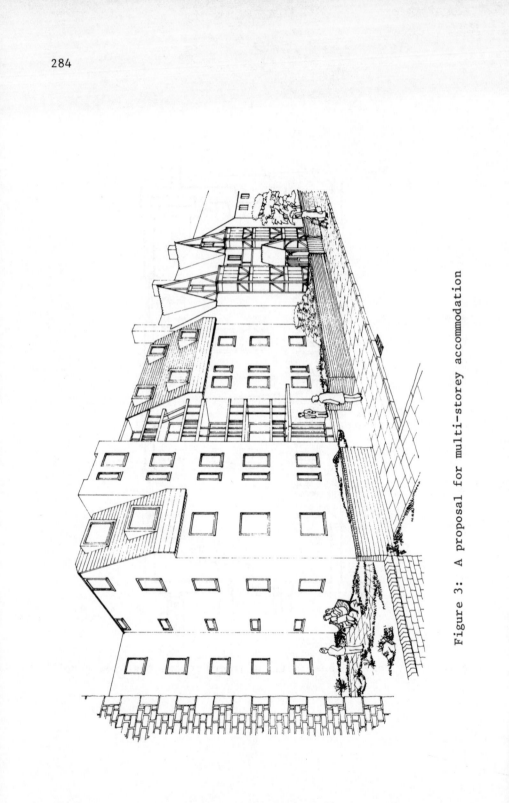

Figure 3: A proposal for multi-storey accommodation

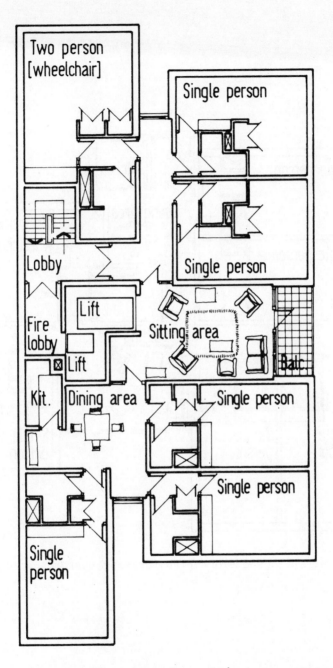

Figure 4: Proposed floor-plan for multi-storey accommodation

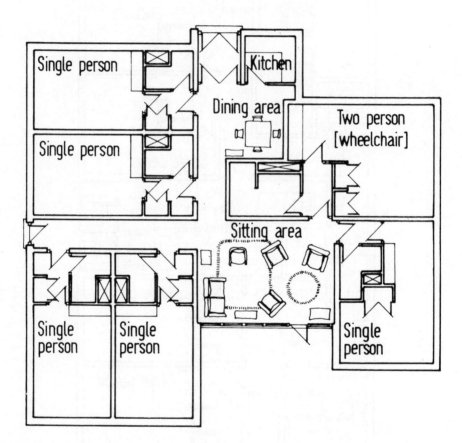

Figure 5: Proposed floor-plan for single storey accommodation

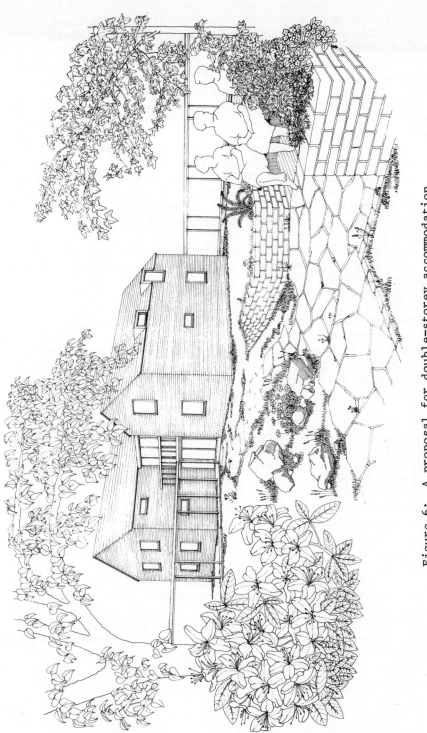

Figure 6: A proposal for double-storey accommodation

For these reasons the proposed designs exclude centralized accommodation of the type shown in Figure 1; namely,
the recommended communal sitting rooms and dining areas
(Ministry of Health, 1962 and 1973). These, we found, readily subject the occupants to staff surveillance and attention. Nor have we provided specifically designed spaces
for non-resident, externally initiated programmes of activity
of the sort advocated by, for instance, Donahue (1964) and
Shore (1964). Whatever their advantages, in our view these
programmes (e.g. preparing and printing mimeographed weekly
news-sheets) reflect and endorse the passive roles assigned
to residents in terms of the hotel model. As their advocates
themselves note, rather than directly harnessing residents'
self-maintenance skills, therapy programmes of this order
tend to rely on sustained intervention by outsiders.

Consistent with the intention of countering an hotel
'image', we have sacrificed large communal areas, e.g. dining
rooms for thirty-two people (Figure 1) and lounges for
twenty-three (Figure 2), in favour of smaller, dispersed,
accommodation. In addition, we have exceeded the recommended
sizes for single and two-person bedrooms, 10 and 15.5 square
metres respectively (Ministry of Health, 1973). The purpose
of this is to provide spaces and facilities that will enable
residents to engage in the day-to-day activities customarily
involved in preparing for sleep, toileting and bathing,
preparing and eating food, and socializing.

Gunzburg and Gunzburg (1973) have furnished an apt
framework for considering the detailed implications of these
intentions. Elaborating their recommendations for developing and maintaining appropriate levels of functioning among
mentally handicapped young people, they urged that suitable
opportunities for activity be made available. To this end,
they argued for physical settings that can be used as "tools"
for experiencing "complete activity cycles". Taking the
daily activity of eating as a case in point, they described
such a cycle:

"...eating must not merely come to mean chewing food
and swallowing it in a socially acceptable form, but must
be associated with shopping, preparing food, cooking, laying
the table, serving, washing hands, washing dishes, clearing
away, cleaning the kitchen, washing tea towels, using washing
powder, hanging up towels for drying, taking them down,
ironing them and putting them into a cupboard till required
again".

As well as illustrating the types and levels of activity
we envisage, this detailed outline highlights the deficiencies we noted whilst working as quasi care attendants during
the participant observation stages of our studies. Dining,
we found, conformed to the hotel service notion. None of
the routines mentioned above were carried out by residents;
the act of choosing food was confined to selecting items
served to them at dining tables. Bathing, dressing for bed
or on waking, and even toileting took place at prescribed
times with, especially in the case of bathing, staff in
attendance. Bedrooms – designated on the architects' draw-
ings and referred to by staff as bedsitting rooms – were,
in the main, only used for sleeping; partially, we were
informed, to allow staff to clean and tidy them. And since
the residents spent most of their waking hours in 'their'
chairs in the communal sitting rooms, conversations tended
to occur among those in immediately neighbouring seats
(Lipman, 1967, and Harris et al, 1977). Consequently, social
exchanges, particularly those with affective content, tended
to be limited to members of dyads or triads considered com-
patible by the staff who had directed the residents to the
chairs they then occupied habitually.

Considering their lifelong experiences, it seems reasonable to presume that at least some of the activities comprising these everyday cycles fall within residents' capabilities. And considering the adverse physiological and
emotional effects that have been attributed to inactivity
in old age (e.g. Bromley, 1974), staff shortages apart,
opportunities for residents to participate appear in and of
themselves to be desirable.

Privacy

From the various definitions of this concept that are
available (e.g. Altman, 1975), we have opted for a socially
rather than an individually orientated formulation; one
suited to congregate living conditions. In the course of a
somewhat complex argument, Bates (1964) claimed that privacy
might most simply be described as:

"...a person's feeling that others should be excluded
from something which is of concern to him, and also a recognition that others have a right to do this".

This view assumes that the value placed on privacy is
shared. It posits some minimum degree of consensus; an
agreement usually associated with the social integration,

or cohesion, held to characterize community-like collectivities (see, for instance, Suttles, 1972).

For Bates then, privacy is, as it were, the obverse of
sociability. Without the shared, the normative, understand-
ings that flow from communal social relations, the concept
has little social meaning. In this sense, the two notions
are inseparable; the one can scarcely be conceived without
invoking the other. If the tensions of collective life are
to be managed, or accommodated, then, the argument runs,
rights to personal and group privacy are to be both recognized and exercised. Access to privacy, in other words,
can be regarded as a buffer between the pressures met in
everyday social intercourse and people's abilities to manage
them.

In our view, the relevance of this argument to the
experience of shared living in Homes is immediate and central. If, as intended (Ministry of Health, 1950), the
experience is to approximate the solidarity of the community
ideal, the privacy of those who occupy them must be recognized and allowed scope for being exercised. And the more
so since such approximations appear unattainable in institutional settings; since the already fragile cohesion of
their fortuitous, merely nominal nature as collectivities
is threatened by the uneven, the divisive, distribution of
authority between staff and residents.

These rights should be extended to all the parties concerned - to resident and staff groups and sub-groups, and
to each individual. Given the stresses of congregate living,
all are likely to require opportunities to be private as
well as public. In formulating our design proposals however,
attention has centred on efforts to enhance residents' opportunities. It is they who are at risk. As Meacher (1972)
noted, prior to being admitted to Homes, it is their views
of personal autonomy that, in most instances, have been
undermined by being defined as requiring residential 'care
and attention'. And once in, it is their privacy that tends
to be jeopardized by the institutional circumstances they
encounter; by, chiefly, staff intrusions into and control
of their daily activities (e.g. Brocklehurst, 1974). Once
in, our studies indicate (Harris, 1978), it is their enforced
social contacts with staff and fellow residents that call
for buffers.

Again we confront the quandary mentioned earlier. How,
in staffed and congregate living situations, can resident
privacy be fostered and maintained? How can the effects of

this contradiction, an apparently inherent contradiction of institutional life (Bennett, 1964), be mitigated?

In lieu of excluding care attendant staff completely, we anticipate that their influence can be minimized most effectively by limiting the range and scope of resident/ staff contacts; by attempting to maximize resident initiative. Although, as compared with changes in the authority relationships prevailing in Homes, physical design can only contribute marginally to such a state of affairs, this seems insufficient grounds on which to discount its potential for providing appropriate physical settings. Appropriate, that is, in that they enhance opportunities for residents to exercise choice vis-à-vis their social contacts. For this reason our proposals seek to separate resident accommodation from major areas of staff activity, to decentralize residents' dining and sitting accommodation, and to facilitate resident self-reliance by making readily available amenities such as personal toilets, showers, and dining spaces. Additionally, with reference to resident/resident contacts, our efforts have been directed to presenting opportunities for solitude as well as company; for individuals and groups to choose independently when and with whom they might seek companionship.

Integration

Our reference to this notion stresses its connotations of "making up of a whole by adding together...separate parts"; in particular, its prosthetic implications of "restoration to wholeness" (Onions, 1972). Accordingly, having attempted to forestall staff aid, we have sought to enable residents to compensate for their deficiencies in carrying out the day-to-day activities mentioned above by calling on the assistance of their peers. Here the intention is to capitalize on the reciprocity involved in exchanges of goods, services and sentiments that anthropologists (e.g. Levi-Strauss, 1964) and sociologists (e.g. Parsons and Shils, 1964) claim is the core of social relations.

Thus, our design proposals depart from current practice whereby so-called confused and rational and, on occasion, physically frail and active elderly people are separately housed (Meacher, 1972). Contrary to present segregationalist policies, our proposals are intended to help affect residential integration. To this end, they comprise grouped accommodation for small numbers of individuals drawn from both these frail and active categories. And to this end, they

include communal as well as personal accommodation in which
reciprocity of services can occur readily among members of
these groupings.

Following his study of three 'confused' and three
'mixed' Homes for old people, Meacher emphasized the advantages of life in integrated venues. The chief benefits for
confused residents, he argued, lie in the aid and stimulation
afforded by the company of their rational co-residents, and
for the latter in the opportunities to take responsibility
for the care of their less able colleagues. (Although he
did not specifically focus on them, it seems reasonable to
anticipate similar advantages from 'integrating' physically
handicapped and active residents.) In so arguing, Meacher
touched on one of the central issues in gerontology: retard-
ing or compensating for the mental, physical and social
deterioration experienced by elderly people, confused,
rational, frail and active alike (Bromley, 1974). Especially
in institutional conditions, it has been claimed that such
retardation or compensation can be assisted by providing
opportunities for maintaining the mental, physical and social
competences residents exercised before entry (e.g. Lawton
and Nahemow, 1973). In Meacher's opinion, opportunities of
this nature, efforts to restore individual 'wholeness' by
drawing on the capabilities of others, are increased in
integrated Homes.

To what extent does integration take place when residents are mixed? Our study of eight Homes sampled, among
other criteria, to maximize the difference in proportions
of confused to rational residents, provided some suggestions.
As reported elsewhere (Harris et al, 1977), we examined two
types of information - locational and interaction data.
Analysis of the former indicated that residents are unlikely
to live in what might be described as a spatially integrated
manner. On the contrary, they can expect to encounter
spatial segregation; if not in their sleeping arrangements,
then by or within the sitting rooms they occupy habitually
and, to a lesser degree, where they take their daily meals.
The interaction data showed a similar trend. Logged recordings of conversations among the three categories of resident
that were identified, the rational, moderately confused and
severely confused, showed, on analysis, that they occurred
primarily within rather than across the categories. Despite
their mixed populations, life in each of the Homes appeared
to be characterized by segregation.

Seeking to account for this situation, we concluded
that it was largely a consequence of the administrative

regimes prevailing in the Homes. Spatial segregation, our participant observation records indicated, had been established and was maintained in order to facilitate the daily services staff administered to residents. And the availability, the ubiquity, of these services contributed to the interactional segregation our analyses disclosed. They remove the grounds on which inter-resident exchanges of services or sentiments might be founded. They precluded reciprocity.

To recapitulate: on three counts, resident activity, privacy and integration, we wish to minimize the institutional dependency implicit in the hotel model of residential care. For this purpose we have referred to another image, a flatlet model: one akin to self-serviced 'digs'-like accommodation for young people (e.g. Allen, 1968), one akin to the notion of 'grouped flatlets' for old people (e.g. Ministry of Housing and Local Government, 1966). However, like merely changing the nomenclature, the changes in built form this model might evoke carry with them no certainty that the relations between those who serve and those who are served will change. As our study indicated (Harris et al, 1977, and Harris, 1978), despite disparate spatial settings the effects of staff-imposed regimes appear to be uniform. Thus we found that resident inactivity was maintained in each of the Homes, on occasion with the aid of drugs. Access to privacy was denied, for instance, by the simple expedient of removing bedroom, bathroom and toilet locks or keys. And·integration was undermined, for example, by demarcating specific bedroom wings, sitting rooms and dining tables on the basis of administrative categorization of residents' mental status.

In these circumstances, assuming a continued demand for residential care and given the untrained status of staff personnel (Personal Social Services Council, 1975), what seems necessary are attempts to limit staff services. While not anticipating that physical design, of itself, will guarantee the success of such efforts, we believe that it can offer a means of facilitating them. As well as providing environments that can support residents' capacities for mutual and self-care, design can help discourage dependence-inducing staff intervention.

THE DESIGN PROPOSALS

Staff/Resident Separation

Complying with the trend in Ministry of Health policies which our colleague Barrett (1976) has traced, we favour 'small' Homes. We accept Korte's (1966) recommendation, founded principally on social grounds, that, where her suggested optimum of twenty-five is exceeded, the number of residents in a Home be limited to approximately forty who are accommodated in 'family groups' of some eight individuals. We do not, however, accept her stipulation that:

"Staff accommodation and facilities should not be strictly separated from residents' accommodation, but should be situated so that residents feel they can have ready access to staff."

In outline, then, our proposals comprise, as a case in point, five single-person bedsitting rooms; each, as well as providing a personal shower and toilet, allowing for the activities involved in the daily cycles of sleeping, sitting, food preparation and eating. Together, with, say, a two-person bedsitting room designed for wheelchair users (see Goldsmith, 1975), these individual rooms are grouped in 'units' that include spaces for group sitting, food preparation and dining. As will be seen from the selected layout plans discussed below, we envisage that such combinations of private bedsitting accommodation and group spaces can be arranged in at least one of three manners. They can form the individual floors of, for instance, a five-storey building (e.g. Figures 3 and 4), they can be detached single-storey units (e.g. Figure 5), or they can take the form of double-storey 'pavilions' consisting of two units (e.g. Figures 6 and 7). In each of these, the units are to be separated from the staff accommodation; access being restricted to stairs and lifts in the former case and to corridor links in the latter two.

These barriers to staff/resident contacts are fundamental to the proposals. They constitute the physical bases of our expectation that, given other propitious factors (such as amenable staff regimens and prosthetic aids for residents), staff services can be limited. We recognize that where most staff or the influential members of staff and/or residents wish to establish and maintain residents' dependence on staff, they will do so. Moreover, as we have noted elsewhere (Harris et al, 1977), they will do so despite apparently inappropriate or inconvenient physical

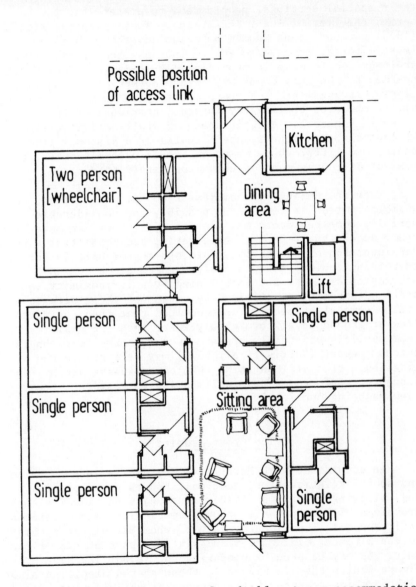

Figure 7: Proposed floor-plan for double-storey accommodation

arrangements. We contend, however, that in negotiating
their spatial settings, people tend to prefer what may be
termed the line of least resistance. Thus, adapting Zipf's
(1965) notions about "human behavior and the principle of
least effort", we have sought to increase the efforts staff
are required to make in providing day-to-day services for
residents. On this count, we favour a vertical, a multi-
storey, arrangement. As the proposed plan indicates (Figure
4), it obviates the lengthy internal corridors of the type
shown in Figure 1. And, if areas of staff activity, such
as centralized kitchens, are situated at a distance from
stairs and lifts, these means of access probably offer the
maximum discouragement of ubiquitous staff attendance.

Notwithstanding our commitment to this separation, we
anticipate that at times, and possibly for considerable
periods, some residents may wish to "feel they can have
ready access to staff". Consequently, and consistent with
our intention of furthering residents' opportunities for
exercising choice, the proposals incorporate a communal
sitting space and a serviced dining area in proximity to
staff accommodation. Limited by virtue of their size to
use by some eight people, we recommend that these be situated at ground level, preferably where they are visible
from publicly accessible areas. Such measures, our observations suggest (Harris et al, 1977) may well reduce the
likelihood of staff confining them to exclusive use by, for
instance, confused or physically disabled residents they
view as being 'unsightly'.

The Grouped Units

In accordance with Korte's (1966) advice on group size
and social relationships, each unit houses seven people.
And following Meacher's (1972) recommendation, ideally these
groupings will comprise a "rough numerical balance" between
frail and able individuals; each of whom has direct access
to the kitchen, dining area and sitting space of his or her
unit. As may be seen by comparing the layout in, say,
Figure 4 with that in Figure 1, these shared amenities highlight a major feature of the proposals; their decentralized
nature.

Apart from hindering the monitoring and surveillance
activities of staff, this dispersed accommodation is intended
to help foster mutual assistance among small groups of residents. Here, in contrast with the hotel-like service
encountered in centralized conditions, those who so desire

can contribute their skills to activity cycles of the type Gunzburg and Gunzburg described in our extract from their recommendations. They can participate in the tasks of preparing, serving and clearing-up after meals: tasks that customarily, our observations indicate, are restricted to members of staff and some two or three 'privileged' residents. Here too, in sitting areas deliberately designed to seat approximately the number in a unit, those who wish to can experience small group sociability. Rather than having to adapt to the institutional, the formal, socio-spatial situations exemplified by the seating arrangements in Figure 2, they can seek companionship in settings of a more domestic, a more informal scale.

These 'social' spaces are supplementary to the analogous but smaller spaces provided in the residents' personal accommodation. And it is to this aspect of the proposals that attention now turns - to the schematic bedsitting room layouts represented by the selected examples in Figures 8 and 9.

The Bedsitting Rooms

With the individual shower cubicles, w.c.'s and lobbies shown on the two sets of plans, the private food preparation, eating and sitting areas in the bedsitting rooms are intended to serve two related purposes. First, in prosthetic terms, they should support residents' efforts to care for themselves. Second, they should help counter the institutional effects of traditionally designed Homes.

Fitted with appropriate aids (e.g. movable hand-operated sprays, slatted seats and grab-rails - Goldsmith, 1976), shower cubicles seem more likely to lend themselves to independent use by elderly people than bathtubs do. Showers can be negotiated by those frail or disabled residents who require help in getting in or out of baths, and are convenient for use by those for whom incontinence necessitates frequent washing without undressing fully. With the similarly equipped toilet compartments, their provision as personal amenities should minimize routine, time-tabled, bathing and toileting by staff. Even if this does not occur, rather than being acknowledged communally, as evidenced by the queues we observed outside centralized bath and toilet blocks, these services need not be administered openly. They can take place in the privacy of residents' personal quarters: a privacy which, we anticipate, will be enhanced by the individual entrances, the domestic 'hall-like' quality afforded by the lobbies.

298

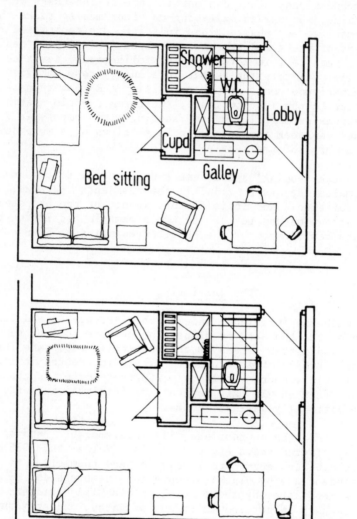

Figure 8: Proposed plan for a wide-front single person bedsitting room showing alternate furniture layouts

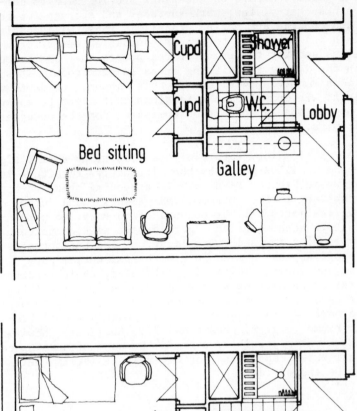

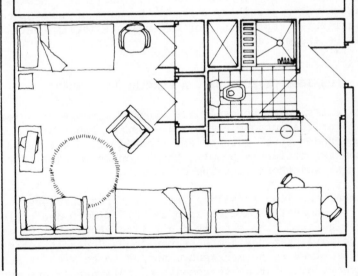

Figure 9: Proposed plan for a narrow-front two person bedsitting room showing alternate furniture layouts

The galleys marked on the plans are intended to comprise sinks, hot-plates, work-surfaces and storage for foodstuff and cooking and eating utensils. These will enable residents independently to prepare snacks or meals for themselves and for the two or three guests they can accommodate in the dining and sitting areas in each room. Thus, as well as receiving visitors in this manner, residents will be able to withdraw from the tensions that might be engendered by the shared activities envisaged for the occupants of the units.

The final major feature of the bedsitting room design we propose is illustrated by the alternative furniture layouts shown in Figures 8 and 9. In stressing this, we hope that, contrary to the uniform arrangements found during our studies, residents will be encouraged to vary, to personalize, their accommodation. Here we are seeking to counter the homogeneity imposed, we believe, by the nursing attention which staff appear to associate with residential care (Kosberg and Gorman, 1975); in particular, their tendency to insist on permitting access to three sides of all beds. To this end, we recommend that units be formed by combining what we have termed 'wide-front' and 'narrow-front' bedsitting rooms (e.g. Figures 8 and 9). Above all, however, we urge wherever possible, even in the case of nursing care, that residents' capacities for actively assisting their fellows be exploited.

POSSIBLE OBJECTIONS - A CONCLUDING COMMENT

Patently, our proposals are open to a range of objections. For the purpose of this discussion these will be subsumed under three categories: those dealing with the preferences of elderly people; those concerned with the buildings; and those centring on staff.

Among the issues falling into the first category, we expect to encounter comment such as "old people don't like living high" and "the elderly don't like showers". Or we might be told that residents prefer to be dependent on staff, to be inactive, to be segregated and/or to be without access to privacy. Insofar as statements of this nature are amenable to being tested empirically, the evidence of which we are aware is ambiguous. For instance, on the question of 'living high' surveys conducted by Hole (1961) and by the Department of the Environment (1975) indicate that, while "the bungalow is still seen as the ideal", respondents are "not deterred by living off the ground" (Todd, 1975).

Lawton, Nahemow and Teaff (1975) on the other hand, report
higher levels of satisfaction among the occupants of 'low
buildings' than those expressed by high-rise dwellers. Despite this, in interpreting their findings, they argue that:

"...high-rise is less familiar to this generation's
elderly and may constitute a psychological barrier...however
(our data)...enable one to conclude that the necessity for
high-rise...should not veto the choice of a particular building...(for old people). Rather, a recognition of the problems...should lead to counteractive administrative efforts
to reduce the possible negative efforts of high-rise on some
tenants".

Criticism levelled at the form of our preferred proposal, the multi-storey building, will, we anticipate, focus
on the issues of cost and escape in the event of fire.
Clearly, a response to the former calls for comparative
analyses of the capital, administrative and maintenance costs
of Homes built on present patterns and those we advocate
(e.g. Hutton, 1975). Indeed, a quantity surveyor's estimate
of the cost of a building based on the proposals indicates
that it falls within the current (1976) cost yardstick.
And an analysis of the revenue consequences of staffing
suggest that the additional capital outlay occasioned by
the increased area of the accommodation we recommend can be
recouped within ten years by the reduced staff complement
called for by the proposals. Further, we believe that, in
view of the possible closure of Homes resulting from constrained economic conditions of the type forecast for the
immediate future (see The Sunday Times, November 23rd, 1975,
p.4), such comparisons should take into account the potential
for wider use our proposals offer. Here we have in mind
their prospects for occupation as 'digs' by, say, nurses,
apprentices or students; that is as types of occupancy for
which, without extensive modification, the accommodation
shown in Figure 1 appears to be unsuited. On the score of
fire: though recognizing the potential hazards, we share
Gunzburg and Gunzburg's (1973) and the Personal Social
Services Council's (1975) opposition to rigidly enforced
regulations that seek to eliminate all risk. With the
Council, we hold that:

"...there is considerable tension between ensuring the
safety yet promoting the freedom of people in care...greater
emphasis may be placed on the avoidance of risks than on
the promotion of high standards of residential life...
Inevitably some risks do have to be taken".

Finally, on the impact or influence of administrative regimens, objections will probably echo our concerns about the tendency of organizational factors to override spatial constraints. Of themselves, the latter are unlikely to secure resident activity, privacy or integration. Indeed, in each of these spheres we expect changes in administrative practices consequent on staff shortages to be more influential. At best our proposals may facilitate such changes. At worse, they may provide the conditions for continuing present practices in Homes; for example, differential allocation to units on the basis of administratively designated mental status (Harris et al, 1977). But even in the latter event, we believe that residents are unlikely to be less advantageously placed than those in the traditionally designed and administered Homes we studied. At minimum, our proposals will increase the range of possibilities open to them.

FOOTNOTE

[1] The discussion in this paper arises from a study supported by a grant (Ref. No. HR2548) awarded to the authors by the Social Science Research Council.

REFERENCES

AGE CONCERN (1973) Age concern on accommodation: views on the problems of housing, with comments by the elderly, National Old People's Welfare Council, London.

ALLEN, P. (1968) "Accommodation for young people", Architects Journal, 147, pp.847-854.

ALTMAN, I. (1975) The environment and social behavior: privacy, personal space, territory, crowding, Brooks/ Cole, Monterey.

ANDERSON, J. E. (1963) "Environment and meaningful activity", in R. H. Williams, C. Tibbits, and W. Donahue (eds.) Processes of aging, Vol.1, Atherton, New York.

BARRETT, A. N. (1976) User requirements in purpose-built local authority residential homes for old people - the notion of domesticity in design, Ph.D. dissertation submitted in the University of Wales.

BARTON, R. (1966) Institutional neurosis, John Wright & Sons, Bristol.

BATES, P. A. (1964) "Privacy - a useful concept?", Social Forces, 42, pp.429-434.

BENNETT, R. G. (1964) "The meaning of institutional life", in M. Leeds, and H. Shore (eds.) Geriatric institutional management, Putnam's, New York, pp.68-91.

BENNETT, R. and NAHEMOW, L. (1965) "Institutional totality and criteria of social adjustment in residences for the aged", Journal of Social Issues, 21, pp.44-78.

BROCKLEHURST, J. C. (1974) Old people in institutions - their rights, Age Concern, London.

BROMLEY, D. B. (1974) The psychology of ageing, Penguin, Harmondsworth.

COMMITTEE ON LOCAL AUTHORITY AND ALLIED PERSONAL SERVICES (Seebohm Report) (1968) Report, Cmd. 3703, H.M.S.O., London.

DEPARTMENT OF THE ENVIRONMENT (1975) The social effects of living off the ground, Housing Development Directorate Occasional Papers 1/75, The Department, London.

DONAHUE, W. (1964) "Restoration and preservation of personality", in M. Leeds and H. Shore (eds.) Geriatric institutional management, Putnam's, New York, pp.186-201

GOLDSMITH, S. (1975) "Wheelchair housing", Architects Journal, 161, pp.1319-1348.

GOLDSMITH, S. (1976) Designing for the disabled, Royal Institute of British Architects, London.

GOFFMAN, E. (1961) Asylums: essays on the social situation of mental patients and other inmates, Doubleday, New York.

GUNZBURG, H. C. and GUNZBURG, A. L. (1973) Mental handicap and physical environment: the application of an operational philosophy to planning, Bailliere Tindall, London.

HARRIS, H. (1978) Maintenance of social order in old people's homes, with special reference to spatial behaviour, M.Sc. dissertation to be submitted in the University of Wales.

HARRIS, H., LIPMAN, A. and SLATER, R. (1977) "Architectural design: the spatial location and interactions of old people", Gerontology, 23, pp.390-400.

HOLE, V. (1961) "Some aspects of housing for old people", Architects Journal, 133, pp.583-586 and 605-608.

HUTTON, K. M. "The cost of sheltered housing as compared with other kinds of residential care", in The role of sheltered housing in the care of the elderly: a re-appraisal, Institute of Social Welfare, Stafford, pp.5-10.

KASTENBAUM, R. (1965) "Theories of human aging: the search for a conceptual framework", Journal of Social Issues, 21, pp.13-36.

KORTE, S. (1966) "Designing for old people: the role of residential homes", Architects Journal, 144, pp.987-991.

KOSBERG, J. I. and GORMAN, J. F. (1975) "Perceptions toward the rehabilitation potential of institutionalized aged", Gerontologist, 15, pp.398-403.

LAWTON, M. P. (1970) "Planning environments for older people", Journal of the American Institute of Planners, 36, pp.124-129.

LAWTON, M. P. (1974) "Research in environmental design for deprived user groups", Journal of Architectural Research, 3, pp.51-54.

LAWTON, M. P. and NAHEMOW, L. (1973) "Ecology and the aging process", in C. Eisdorfer and M. P. Lawton (eds.) The psychology of adult development and aging, American Psychological Association, Washington.

LAWTON, M. P., NAHEMOW, L. and TEAFF, J. (1975) "Housing characteristics and the well-being of elderly tenants in federally assisted housing", Journal of Gerontology, 30, pp.601-607.

LEVI-STRAUSS, C. (1964) "The principle of reciprocity", in L. A. Coser, and B. Rosenberg (eds.) Sociological theory: a book of readings, Macmillan, New York, pp.74-84.

LINDSLEY, O. R. (1964) "Geriatric behavioral prosthetics", in R. Kastenbaum (ed.) New thoughts on old age, Springer, New York, pp.41-60.

LIPMAN, A. (1967) "Chairs as territory", New Society, 9, pp.564-566.

LIPMAN, A. (1968) "Some problems of direct observation in architectural social research", Architects Journal, 147, pp.1349-1356.

LIPMAN, A. (1970) "Accommodation for the elderly", in Modern british geriatric care, Whitehall Press, London, pp.423-427.

MASLOW, A. H. (1943) "A theory of human motivation", Psychological Review, 50, pp.370-397; cf. also W. H. Haythorn (1970) "A needs by sources of satisfaction analysis of environmental habitability", Ekistics, 30, pp.200-203.

MEACHER, M. (1972) Taken for a ride, special residential homes for confused old people: a study of separatism in social policy, Longman, London.

MINISTRY OF HEALTH (1950) Report of the Ministry of Health for the year ended 31st March 1949, Cmd. 7910, H.M.S.O., London.

MINISTRY OF HEALTH (1962) Residential accommodation for elderly people, Local Authority Building Note 2, H.M.S.O., London; cf. also Metric Edition, 1973.

MINISTRY OF HOUSING AND LOCAL GOVERNMENT (1966) Old people's flatlets at Stevenage: an account of the project with an appraisal, Design Bulletin 11, H.M.S.O., London.

ONIONS, C. T. (ed.) (1972) The shorter Oxford English dictionary on historical principles, Clarendon Press, Oxford.

PARSONS, T. and SHILS, E. A. (1964) "The basic structure of interactive relationship", in L. A. Coser and B. Rosenberg, (eds.) Sociological theory: a book of readings, Macmillan, New York. pp.84-86.

PASTALAN, L. A. (1970) "Privacy as an expression of human territoriality", in L. A. Pastalan and D. H. Carson (eds.) Spatial behavior of older people, University of Michigan Press, Ann Arbor.

PERSONAL SOCIAL SERVICES COUNCIL (1975) Living and working in residential homes: interim report of a working group, The Council, London.

SCHWARTZ, A. N. (1975) "An observation of self-esteem as the linchpin of quality of life for the aged: an essay", Gerontologist, 15, pp.470-472.

SHORE, H. (1964) "A resident-directed adult study program", in M. Leeds and H. Shore (eds.) Geriatric institutional management, Putnam's, New York, pp.222-226.

SLATER, R. (1968) Adjustment of residents to old age homes, M.Phil. dissertation submitted in the University of Sussex.

SNYDER, L. H. (1973) "An exploratory study of patterns of social interaction, organization, and facility design in three nursing homes", International Journal of aging and Human Development, 4, pp.319-333.

SUTTLES, G. D. (1972) The social construction of communities, University of Chicago Press, Chicago.

TODD, H. (1975) "Research report", Age Concern Today, 15, p.10.

TOWNSEND, P. (1962) The last refuge: a survey of residential institutions and homes for the aged in England and Wales, Routledge & Kegan Paul, London.

TOWNSEND, P. (1975) "Inflation and low incomes", New Statesman, 90, pp.245-247.

TUNSTALL, J. (1966) Old and alone, Routledge & Kegan Paul, London.

ZIPF, G. K. (1965) Human behavior and the principle of least effort: an introduction to human ecology, Hafner, New York.

Evaluating
Acute General Hospitals

CHERYL KENNY AND DAVID CANTER

INTRODUCTION

This chapter considers the evaluation of the design of
acute general hospitals. Of all the building types this
century, acute hospitals has been the one which has grown
most directly out of a series of post-design evaluations
and subsequent modifications of future buildings. In part
this has been due to an awareness of rapid changes in medical
technology. The lessons to be learned by earlier successes
and failures have also been necessary because of the great
cost and complexity of major hospital buildings. This systematic approach to the evolution of design concepts was
influenced greatly by the work of the Nuffield Research Team
led by Llewelyn-Davies (1955), which commenced soon after
World War II. As Stone (1976) points out, before the establishment of this project:

"No study work was being done, or had been done anywhere
in the world at that time, on fundamental problems of hospital planning. Some specific aspects had been studied,
for example by the Medical Research Council in the area of
bacteriology, but there has been little literature on the
general problem of hospital design since Florence Nightingale's
1863 book 'Notes on Hospitals'."

The unique quality of the Nuffield Study was to examine
in a systematic, multi-disciplinary way what actually happen-
ed in hospitals and the likely implications for design of
proposed nursing and medical policies. Wherever possible
measurements were made and predictive models developed. But
of probably greatest significance was the fact that the
Nuffield Team converted their findings into designs and

illustrated their research report with plans for proposed wards.

Stone (1976) charts the development of this line of research and shows how it led from a consideration of ward design, which was the major contribution of the Nuffield Project, to the development of an approach to general layout of hospital buildings, on the basis of communication networks. This later evolved into an approach to hospital design which dealt with the complex of structural and service systems as a unity. Each of these stages of development was preceded by a variety of research activity usually supported by the Department of Health and Social Security. Surprisingly, it was rare in this research for the patients' views and experiences to be given much weight. In retrospect it would seem that the dominant perspective, of seeing the problem as a technological one, led to a concern for the strengths and weaknesses of the existing building layout and hardware. It was only when the new generation of buildings which emerged from this research was actually being used that management and designers became concerned to learn how the staff and patients in these buildings made use of them and felt about them.

The impetus for considering user reactions to hospital design has been given further force by the growing criticism of the 'medical model' on which hospital practice is founded. The criticism is led by medical sociologists (see Stacey, 1977, for a review). They see the general hospital as the focal point of this 'medical model' because it is geared to the treatment of individual illness and pathology. Such a model, they suggest, prevents intervention before symptoms occur, treats illness not whole persons, places the onus on the professionals to maintain a healthy society rather than on the individual and is a result of the professionals' unwillingness to share their control and responsibilities with the wider community. They argue that a major shift in orientation would be of value so that the entire community would become the therapeutic environment with the aim of prevention top priority (through education, better housing, etc.).

Of particular design relevance in the criticism of the medical model is the dependency of patients on the professionals and their elaborate technological support systems. From an environmental design point of view, therefore, it is possible to see the medical model as an example of what Burton et al. (1968) have called a 'technological fix'.

Burton and his colleagues used this term with reference to national policies towards potential natural hazards (e.g. flood, hurricanes etc.). The essence of this attitude is that technology can be applied to prevent disaster from striking. The result of this approach is that people do not consider their individual actions as contributory to the probability of a disaster occurring (for example where they choose to live) and consequently feel no responsibility for modifying their actions. They see both the cause and cure outside of their control. A similar situation exists with respect to health and illness. The contraction of illness is generally seen as 'bad luck' and expected treatment is in the form of later intervention of the professionals' technology. This implies that the general hospital, with its operating theatres, medical wards and its many other facilities, not only makes a 'technological fix' possible, it also symbolises it.

An evaluation of a hospital is, as a consequence, inevitably an exploration of the way in which doctors and nurses see the hospital supporting their professional role and symbolising that support. An evaluation is also an investigation of the reactions of patients to those symbolic and support qualities.

This paper explores the assessment, made by the various groups within the hospital, of the relationship between the physical setting and the goals of the practitioners and patients. It commences by looking at hospitals as a whole, then progresses to consider those areas where patients have their most direct contact with the system, the Hospital Ward.

EVALUATING WHOLE HOSPITALS

One of the major pieces of work on patients' views of their acute general hospitals is that of Raphael (1969) which identified three broad categories of patient concern; care of the patient, the physical environment and life in hospital. On the whole, patients were remarkably satisfied with their experience in hospital. In response to the question "Have you found the hospital satisfactory in its care of patients?" 73% replied "very satisfied".

Of further interest in Raphael's work, with respect to the evaluation of the whole hospital, are the differences between the staff and the patients and between staff who have differing responsibilities. In respect to the above question about patient care, the staff were far less enthusiastic about their hospitals. The percentage of doctors, nurses and administrators which considered this care very satisfactory were 21, 29 and 23 per cent respectively. This is not particularly surprising as the staff would be better acquainted with the potential quality of care that was possible. Also, more importantly, these percentages disguise the particular aspect of the hospital to which each group was referring. In analysis of a further question "If I could alter one thing..." (Raphael 1965), there were found to be considerable differences between the groups in what they thought should be given top priority for change. The patients wanted change with respect to life in the hospital, such as food, ways of passing the time and the social environment. The major priority category for the staff, this includes the doctors, nurses, administrators and committee members, was the physical environment. When the groups were compared on specific suggestions, the nurses were most similar to the patients, while there was little or no agreement between the patients and the doctors and committee members (the two groups which most probably have the greatest amount of control over the hospital). In response to reports returned to hospitals, the recommendations which were most frequently adopted were those to do with the physical environment.

Organisational Roles

To assess the contribution the physical environment makes in helping (or hindering) the goals of the hospital, requires knowledge of the particular hierarchies that exist in the organisation of the hospital, and an understanding of how the various groups conceptualise the physical environment with respect to their goals. Green (1974), for example, demonstrates that there are twelve different major groups at work within a typical hospital, excluding the administration. Each of these has a distinct hierarchical organisation. Canter's (1972) study of a large district hospital for children helps demonstrate the significance of this. He compared the evaluations of a wide group of users. Unfortunately he was unable to obtain comparable results from the patients, who were mainly young children, but he was able to show that the administrators, doctors and nursing staff each had characteristically different evaluations. These differences clearly related to their goals and the extent to which their roles depended upon technological support systems, the consultants, for example, being much happier with the new cardiology and intensive care facilities than any other groups; the administrators being relatively happiest with the dining facilities and the nursing staff warming to the non-clinical setting for the child and family psychiatry unit.

This study was also unusual in using the process of evaluation to look back into the design and production of the hospital, including a detailed examination of the conceptualisations of those individuals who had had major roles in designing and managing the hospital. This revealed the way in which many of the later strengths and weaknesses of the hospital were a function of the constraints under which the design was produced and the cognitive system upon which the designers drew for their design concepts. Analysis of 'repertory grid' responses from the architect indicated that the architect considered places where patients were and places with high medical involvement to be in opposition, suggesting that he had a rather oversimplified notion of patient and staff contacts. In other words, the impact of prior research findings, design guidelines or any other 'scientific' literature can only operate against a background of psychological preconceptions. In many cases these pre-existing states can mask the effect of any 'new' material. (See Canter, 1977, for a detailed review of these issues.) It could be suggested that the major gap in information for design is not in technological data, but systematic accounts of what people actually do in a given place and how they conceptualise the physical environment with respect to those activities.

Location and Role

One of the few studies which has attempted to investigate directly the relationship between the organisational structure of a hospital and the physical setting is Rosengren and De Vault's (1963) informal observation of an obstetrical hospital. This setting has two main advantages in terms of such work. Firstly, it has a very definite medical goal - childbirth. Secondly, it has a limited and very well defined sequence of places through which the patient moves as she progresses through various stages of childbirth. The two work groups were doctors and the nurses, each with their own hierarchical structure. The official organisational structure was easily identifiable by the quality and provision of space for private use. The consultant's lounge was well appointed and near the centre of the unit; the interns' lounge was more peripheral and adjacent to a laboratory and austere in appearance, while only meagre provision was available to the student nurses.

The main interest for this work lies in the analysis of the areas through which the patient moved. It was possible to identify shifts in status which occurred for the professional as well as the patient in the various places, and the physical characteristics of these places which help to facilitate this.

Ultimate control of the Unit was maintained by the consultants and administrative nurses. However, the spaces that they actively controlled were the delivery room and adjacent theatre, which were the most central areas in the Unit. Here was the greatest display of hospital trappings (bright lights, uniforms, etc.). Peripheral to this area were the reception, 'prep', labour and recovery rooms. Each room that the women passed through was segregated from the rest. This segregation helped to facilitate the informal but accepted structure of control. One instance was the labour room which was screened by shoulder height barriers and was the province of the nurses. Within this space the status allotted the interns was dependent upon whether or not a patient was present. If the nurses would be overheard by a patient, they addressed the interns as Dr., otherwise they only referred to them by last names, thus emphasising that they, the interns, did not really belong in that place.

This setting, then, is characterised by (a) the spatial segregation of the areas of control and (b) the role norms related to the hierarchical structure of the organisation and the area of the hospital. For example, nurses were very reluctant to venture an opinion in the operating theatre. These two characteristics may facilitate the functioning of the specific areas but could be detrimental to the functioning of the hospital as a whole. The difficulties of communication between these rigid organisation structures is endorsed by the work of Coser (1958). She demonstrated that when information must move up the nursing hierarchy and down that of the medical people, it not only delays decision making, but affects the degree to which the nurses feel involved in the system.

In the obstetrical hospital this problem resulted in a totally different set of role norms developing, for the only place which did not have clearly defined control, the corridor. Here, opinions could be and were expressed without threat to the individual reputation.

The final interesting aspect of the obstetrical hospital was the close relationship between the attitudes of the professional towards the patient and her actual location within the hospital. These professional attitudes were defined by the contribution the patient was making to the overall goal - childbirth. There appeared to be only two

areas where the patient had active roles. In the reception
area she was still a person. The open design of the place
and informal dress of those in charge led to a welcoming
atmosphere. The only other place where she had a definite
role was in the delivery room. The other rooms the patient
moved through were physically peripheral to the delivery
room, drab in appearance and manned by persons of lower
status. These were the 'prep', labour and recovery rooms.
The attitudes towards the patients in these rooms were most
clearly demonstrated by how 'pain' was handled. In the
delivery room pain was considered legitimate because it
directly contributed to the overall goal and relieving pain
could become an additional goal because the 'technological
fix' solution was available in the person of the anaes-
thetist. Such technology was not available in the other
rooms and pain was either dismissed as a nuisance or handled
by emotional support from the lower status professionals.

The Hospital as an Industrial Complex

The literature we have discussed here points in a rather
unexpected direction. Raphael's work pointed to the differing views of the hospital users, Canter demonstrates how
these views led to a very different assessment of the success
of the hospital design and Rosengren and DeVault observed
that the layout of the hospital may accentuate these user
group differences. Once the user's perspective is used in
the evaluation of hospitals, instead of taking solely the
'experts' evaluation of a technological system which the
Nuffield and earlier research had done, one of the major
weaknesses of the medical model and its associated technological fix becomes apparent. This model appears to stimulate
a highly fractionated and diverse set of group goals and
consequent group requirements. The hospitals which emerge
from the studies described do not seem to be coherent communities with common goals for provision of patient care.
Instead they seem to be industrial complexes housing a number
of separate processes, each with its own set of skilled
operations and each with its own criteria for evaluating the
success of its product. The patient, sometimes literally,
is moved from department to department to be subjected to
the relevant technology. Clearly the sophisticated operations,
procedures and equipment which are considered essential for
any modern hospital are not the only cause, nor necessarily
a direct cause, of the fragmentation which characterises a
large acute hospital, but they must surely be a significant
contribution.

EVALUATING HOSPITAL WARDS

The rich variety which constitutes a hospital is probably less apparent to a patient than it is to researchers. If the patient is taken as the 'focal' person in the total setting then the ward must be considered the most critical setting. Life in hospital for the patient, as demonstrated by Raphael, is centred upon the ward in which they are, with the most important user groups for the patient being nurses and the other patients.

The review of the historical development in ward design, presented in the Nuffield Report (1955), illustrated that the changes in layout, size and facilities that had occurred in the early years of hospital building were directly related to the stage of development of the medical profession.

It would seem that at the turn of the eighteenth century complicated surgery was not possible and for the most part the role of the wards was to provide care rather than treatment. From writings of the time comes the impression that they were generally informal, relaxed places without the rigid routine that was to later characterise the hospital ward. Alkin (1771) and Howard (1791), authorities on hospitals at that time, both discussed the provision of small wards with good circulation of air and provision of sitting rooms to aid convalescence.

By the mid-nineteen hundreds anaesthesia had changed the character of wards. The more sophisticated surgical procedures that were possible increased the amount of clinical treatment given to patients. The recommended procedure was that patients spend a long time with complete bed rest to avoid opening a wound. This changed the responsibilities of the nurses considerably. They not only needed greater skills to attend to the patients, but also a ward design that would allow maximum surveillance of the patients while they were in bed. At this time, the most authoritative writer on ward design and function was Florence Nightingale. She considered the two most important criteria for determining the number of beds and nurses on a ward were "ease of supervision and economy of attendance" (1863). Up until this time the average number of patients looked after by a sister and two nurses was twenty. She calculated that with adequate supplies of hot and cold water and lifts, this number could be increased to thirty-two. The result of these recommendations and the necessity for economy was the 30-bedded open plan ward which still carries her name.

While a very large percentage of wards in use in Britain are still open plan, the debate between the building of open plan as opposed to partitioned wards rarely arises. Since World War II nearly all plans sub-divide wards into 4-6 bedded bays or rooms. The impetus for smaller, partitioned wards came from the continent and the United States. The Nuffield Report suggested that the adoption of this ward form was due to increased concern about patient comfort and for the possibility of a higher occupancy of beds (either by mixing specialities or sexes within a ward).

The major criteria for ward design (as presented by the Nuffield Report Building Evaluation 1955) is for <u>maximum</u> economy, <u>proper</u> conditions for medical care, and <u>adequate</u> amenities for the patient.

How these requirements are accommodated in the partitioned wards is no longer totally dependent upon the developments in the medical profession. For example, Florence Nightingale requested only hot and cold water to facilitate the work of the nurses. Now, as suggested by Stone (1976) one of the major impacts on ward design has been the vast increase in equipment for automating the supply and disposal systems used in hospitals.

In addition, there are now many policies which must be considered in designing new wards and hospitals. Noakes (1971) in his review of ward planning lists several issues which directly affect the ward design. They are:

(a) progressive patient care

(b) mixing specialities within wards

(c) the pattern of nursing management

(d) the number of beds per ward, per room and per nursing station

(e) the function of the nurses' station

(f) the number of single rooms requested for each ward

(g) increased concern about the relationship between the individual ward and the whole hospital

This review of the development of ward design in
Britain is not intended to be comprehensive, but rather to
demonstrate the variety of issues which must be taken into
account during the decision making stages in the design of
hospitals, and in particular, wards. If evaluation is
taken to mean not a description of the contents, but an
assessment of the success of the design in terms of those
who use it, given the complexity of modern requirements,
what is the most fruitful approach to evaluation in order
to facilitate this decision making process?

Patients and their Wards

One objective of the Nuffield research was to establish
the number of patients who could be served by a particular
facility. For certain facilities the criterion was the
frequency of use and straightforward assessments were possible e.g. the utility rooms. However, for other facilities
categorisation of the patients had to be established before
realistic deductions could be made. The first of these was
in relation to the location and number of single rooms
which should be provided. It was necessary to determine
what type of patient would be likely to use these. The
criterion for this was obtained from 24 specialities who
provided five different categories of patients. These were
grouped into two general categories: patients who need close
attention and patients, although not needing close observation, who could not be kept in multi-bedded rooms. Using
this category system doctors on 24 wards daily assessed the
number of patients who would qualify for the use of the
single room if it were available. From this data, it is
possible to establish a mathematical model for a given ward
size and speciality of the most appropriate number of single
rooms and their location, to balance efficiency of provisions (the percentage of patients requiring single rooms)
and the efficiency of use (the percentage of patients using
the room).

This research demonstrates the possibility of defining
and clarifying general policies through research which are
instrumental in forming the final design solution. They
also provided the basis for the later evaluation of the
finished product. At Musgrave Park (Nuffield, 1962) one of
the two hospitals which built their wards on the Nuffield
design, records were kept for two years on the percentage
of people using facilities. This made it possible to make
direct comparisons with the predictions established in the
earlier research. The major deficiency of this work is

that the views of the actual user under consideration, the patient, was not seen as an essential element in formulating the policies. If the objective is to provide a therapeutic environment a clear understanding of what that setting means to the client is necessary.

Since the work of the Nuffield Trust was conducted, many 'patient opinion' surveys have been carried out to identify the aspects of ward design which are of concern to the patient (Cartwright, 1964; Waters and MacIntyre, 1977; Raphael, 1969; Wilson-Barnett, 1976; Eardley and Wakefield, 1973; Tranter, 1977; Hicks, 1976). The findings from these 'polls' show considerable consistency in the sources of dissatisfaction for patients with respect to characteristics of the physical design. The one most frequently criticised feature within the ward was the sanitary facilities. These were criticised in terms of provision, condition and lack of privacy within these facilities.

Noise levels were also considered to be a problem, particularly noise from other patients. The noise from other patients and staff was seen as particularly acute at night time. The problem of noise can be considered part of a more general issue, lack of privacy for the patient. Within the ward, patients found control of information about themselves most difficult when trying to have discussions with staff and visitors and when being treated (both medical treatment and when being tended, e.g. use of the bedpan). The fourth aspect of the physical environment most frequently criticised was the heating and ventilation, with the majority of complaints suggesting wards were too hot and stuffy. The most striking similarity between these four aspects is that they can all be grouped together as a statement of 'lack of control, by patients, of their environment'.

All these studies have identified issues which were considered more important to the patients than the physical attributes. The most comprehensive view of a patient's stay in hospital was presented by Raphael (1969). Through the analysis of unstructured interviews in four British hospitals, she identified three broad categories of concern: (a) care of the patient, (b) the physical environment, and (c) life in hospital. These categories and Raphael's sub-categories were also found by Tranter (1969) using a similar method. Within the two categories of care and life in hospital, the majority of the above studies found patients to express concern about obtaining information from the staff about their condition, compatability between patients and the lack of activities which could absorb the long hours spent on the ward.

One aspect which is noticeable in all the work is the gratitude of the patients towards the staff. In particular, the care given by nurses was consistently assessed as the most positive feature of their stay in hospital. Also it must be stated that the frequency of negative comments with regard to all aspects of the hospital stay was, in general, very low, even in wards which were in very poor condition.

The issues which cause concern with respect to the physical and social environment and with the care of the patient all demonstrate the lack of control the patient has over what happens to him. All this fits well with the notion that the 'technological fix' approach to health leads to people having to sacrifice individual control in order for the professional to take responsibility for their treatment. What needs careful consideration is the cost, to the patient, of this dependency. Wilson-Barnett (1976) talks of 'hospital factors' causing distress. The example she quotes is Haywards (1975) demonstration that pre-operative explanation of the surgical procedures to the patient was associated with a decreased need for post-operative analgesia. Wilson-Barnett's own research found that patients not only expressed concern about inadequate information about their condition but also about the lack of information regarding their role as a patient and what was expected of them. Taken as a whole the research described above presents patients as a vulnerable group, and as suggested by Waters and MacIntyre (1977), because patients are prepared to express so few complaints, when they do occur they should be taken very seriously.

From the environmental point of view, this work is frustrating because the physical setting is dealt with as though it were something completely separate from other aspects of being a patient. What is needed is an approach which can integrate the three areas identified by Raphael (care of the patient, the physical environment, and life in hospital) to provide a total description of the experience of being a patient in a hospital.

An initial start has been made by Sears and Auld (1976) in their evaluation of the facilities and design features of acute wards. From loosely structured interviews with ward users about their particular ward, a general questionnaire was developed for use by all people found in a hospital ward (e.g. patients, nurses, visitors, doctors, etc.). The questionnaire contained questions on specific aspects of the ward and a general evaluation measure of the whole ward using bipolar adjectives. The questionnaire was distributed

in 34 wards in 16 hospitals. Of the 1,334 respondents 404
were patients. One of the objectives of this work was to
identify which areas of concern to the patients contributed
most to the general evaluation score given to a ward. They
found that for patients the three areas which contributed
most to the general assessment of the ward were: ease of
surveillance and patients' sense of security, provision of
and privacy within the sanitary facilities and space and
facilities for patients out of bed.

This work is important for two reasons. The first is
that it illustrates that the patients' view of the ward as
a place includes more than just the specific features for
which there are frequent complaints. The second reason is
that the work demonstrates that it is possible to assess
the physical environment in terms of the extent to which it
facilitates care of the patient and contributes to a con-
genial social environment. In fact it suggests that the
greatest impact of the ward on patients is the extent to
which it facilitates the various contacts, both positive
and negative, between patients and staff and among patients.
The 'areas' or factors which contributed most to the general
evaluation of the ward show marked similarities to the concerns expressed by patients, with regard to the care provided
by staff and the social environment, identified in the
studies discussed previously.

The advantage of the ward being the focus for the
patient is that it can become a place of security within
the fragmented hospital complex, but this can be counter-
productive if the ward is so removed as to produce isolation
and/or encourage a highly dependent, passive role for the
patient. Therefore, to gain maximum benefit from the
cocooning qualities of the ward the general recommendations
from the pieces of research summarised here are that the
ward as a place should facilitate contact with the staff to
reduce anxiety while encouraging independence, in order to
enable patients to experience a sense of control over what
is happening to them. Before it will be possible to systematically evaluate various ward designs against these criteria,
greater clarification is needed of the relationship between
on the one hand those activities and goals which make up
the experience of being a patient, and on the other, the
physical organisation of the ward.

Nurses and their Wards

Evaluating ward designs with respect to nursing activities does not present the same problems as those associated

with research relating to patients. The role of the nurse is not ambiguous. Nurses are there to provide nursing care and ward design should facilitate that goal. The question of course is what is nursing care. This paper cannot begin to present a comprehensive analysis of the role of the nurse and must rely upon the definitions provided by the research described below.

Again the first major research relating nursing activities to ward design was the work of the Nuffield Trust (1955). Their objective was to produce a ward design which would maximise nursing efficiency, and facilitate patient centred treatment. The work, orientated towards improved efficiency, consisted of detailed ergonomic studies of nursing procedures at the bedside to determine the most efficient distances between beds, recordings of the nurses' journeys within the ward to provide information on the most appropriate locations of facilities such as the utility rooms within the wards, and also frequency and duration of use of these ancillary facilities to aid in their design.

The other major area of research which was used to formulate their design was the Job Analysis (1953) of nursing in the ward. They found that three quarters of 'nursing' was being carried out by students while the sister and staff nurses were mainly taken up with 'administration'. This was also reflected in their analysis of the pattern of nurses' movements in the ward. It was found that the majority of journeys were from bed to bed and were due to specific nurses carrying out specific tasks for all the patients, these tasks being related directly to the nurse's qualifications. The recommendations made were to assign a limited number of patients to a particular student nurse in order that she would have the opportunity to nurse a whole person. Adjustments made to these recommendations, that trained nurses should nurse and not just supervise, and trained nurses should be in charge of all the nursing of a group of patients, led to the concept of the Nursing Unit. Several of these would make up the Ward, the Administrative Unit.

As stated earlier, the Nuffield project was in the unique position of utilising their research findings to directly influence the production of a ward design. This necessitated a broader approach to ward evaluation than has characterised most recent research. For example both improved efficiency and more patient centred care were seen as design objectives.

The follow up evaluation of Musgrave Park (Nuffield 1962), indicated that the nursing organisation and the layout

of the wards were both successful with the major exception
being the size of the bed bays. Unfortunately this assessment did not maintain the same standards of careful research
which characterised the work leading to the original design
principles. This lack of systematic methods has remained a
problem with the majority of work aimed at evaluating the
success of ward designs. As noted by O'Leary (1975), they
are usually case studies of whole hospitals conducted by
teams of experts. He also indicates that they are often
written up in such a manner as to make it difficult to
generalize to other settings, the methods of gathering
information are informal and they seldom identify exactly
whose impressions are being recorded.

Since the Nuffield study of nurses' journeys within a
ward, much work has been done to produce mathematical models
to predict the amount of movement necessitated by various
ward layouts (Sturdavant, 1960; Thompson, 1959; Freeman and
Smalley, 1968; and Lippert, 1971). The most comprehensive
approach was that of Lippert, 1971, which utilized the previous work to predict, not just the distances between two
locations within the ward, but also the travel distances of
various types of nurse tours (that is, moving through a
series of locations within the ward). These tours could
be, for example, highly ordered with the nurse leaving the
nursing station and visiting each patient in turn or the
tours could be random, visiting patients in an order which
bore no relation to their location within the ward.

The results of the work "showed that the essential
description of nurses' travel as a function of the layout
of the nursing unit could be described by simple algebraic
expressions". This they suggest has implications both for
the architect designing wards and for the organisation of
nursing activities. For example, the work demonstrates
that visiting more patients per tour reduces the total
travel per patient. It appears that work of this nature
assumes that efficiency (defined as distances travelled) is
equated with good nursing care. Such an assumption would
lead to the conclusion that 'assembly line' nursing care
would improve the quality of that care. This is very different from the concept of team nursing as proposed by the
Nuffield Job Analysis (1953) with its emphasis on treating
the patient as a whole person. This is not to deny that
efficient layouts are essential for facilitating good nursing
care, but a fragmented definition of the role of the nurse
can be of only limited value in providing an environment
which will facilitate all the activities and goals which go
to make up nursing care.

Relating Evaluation to Ward Design

A comprehensive approach to the relationship between ward designs and nursing activities is represented by the work of Trites et al (1970). They were provided with the unique opportunity of evaluating wards which were built for the purpose of research. The sample consisted of twelve wards, which varied only in their shape. Three were of the radial design, three were of the double corridor design and three were single corridor wards. The research methods employed were time sampling, recording of nursing activities and their locations and questionnaires on the subjective feelings of the nurses.

Detailed recording of the patients' condition to determine patient-dependency levels in each ward and records of occupancy were also kept in order to control for their possible influences on the activities in the wards. The analysis of the activity data demonstrated that the nurses on the radial wards not only spent less time in travelling around the ward but that this greater efficiency in layout resulted in these nurses spending more time actually with the patients. The analysis of staff absenteeism, staff accidents on the ward, and questions about which type of ward design nurses, doctors and patients preferred, all confirmed the greater success of the radial shaped wards.

Sears and Auld (1976) also explored the relationships between the factors which contributed most to the overall evaluation of the ward and some of the physical variables. They found so many significant correlations that no interpretable pattern could be found in the results. Consequently, forty-four variables relating to floor areas, sanitary facilities, lighting and equipment were selected for further analysis. Separate analyses were conducted for each of the four above groups. This reduced the physical characteristics to eleven component scores for each ward. This data was further simplified by grouping the wards on the basis of the eleven components. From this, five ward types were identified.

It was only at this point of data reduction that meaningful relationships could be established between the two different sets of data, and then only at the most general level. For example, the open-plan Nightingale wards were most successful with respect to ease of surveillance, with the layout of the modern wards being seen as inconvenient.

Through further analysis with respect to the general layout of the ward, Sears and Auld began to illustrate the 'mechanics' of the ward which led to the above general results. They found that when the proportion of beds visible from the nursing station was controlled, the correlation between the evaluation of the wards with respect to surveillance and the physical variable of 'size of the main circulation area' was only significant for the unqualified nursing staff. For the other user groups, if the layout facilitated adequate patient observation the amount of walking necessitated by the design layout did not affect their evaluation of the ward.

This analysis of the relationship between the subjective assessments and the actual design characteristics demonstrates the difficulties which are encountered in such work when no framework or overall model is available to aid in that description. Thus while they were able to demonstrate general relationships, the investigation of the intricate aspects of design were restricted to consideration of only the joint effects of two physical variables with respect to one 'area of concern' or component of the users' subjective experience. It can be proposed that the difficulties arose from the fragmented approach taken to establish the structure of the users' experience of the ward.

An initial step towards a wholistic approach to subjective appraisals is being developed by the authors and their colleagues in the Hospital Evaluation Research Unit, at the University of Surrey, using questionnaires for nurses and patients to evaluate acute wards. This work is similar to that of Sears and Auld (1976) in that the questionnaires were based on interviews with the users and that statistical analysis was used to identify the components which make up the users' experience of the ward. Although the Unit is in the early stages of their research, some very important differences are apparent. Firstly, the questionnaires for patients and for nurses are being developed totally separately. Secondly, these questionnaires have undergone extensive pilottings which have included interviews with the users about the questionnaires to ensure their clarity and validity. However, the most important difference was the incorporation of an approach to the analysis which provides an <u>overview</u> of reactions to hospital wards. This overview is summarised in Table 1. The Table is based on a form of analysis derived from the work of the Israeli Social Scientist, Guttman. But without going into technical details, inappropriate for the present volume, the Table can be explained as a summary of all the possible questions which may be asked of nurses about the design of their ward. Each cell in the Table represents a series of questions. For example,

TABLE 1

A 2-dimensional representation of the 'overview' of reactions
to hospital wards

SOCIAL ASPECT

PLACE	EFFICIENCY	COMFORT
LOCATIONS WITHIN THE WARD	Layout of the bedspace for treatment	Layout of the bedspace for patient privacy Layout of the ward (private place) for staff privacy
THE WARD IN GENERAL	Layout of the ward to move patients/supplies Layout of the ward to observe patients	Layout of the ward for patient companionship/recreation Atmosphere of the ward for comfort

NON-SOCIAL ASPECT

LOCATION	Capacity of storage facilities to store supplies/equipment	Heating/ventilation for patient comfort
WARD	Lighting of the ward for nursing activities	

the top left cell represents questions dealing with nursing efficiency relating to particular locations, such as bed space, on the ward. Besides summarising a broad set of questions the Table itself provides pointers to the key issues of concern to nurses in ward design.

Although this work is still at a very early stage, this preliminary analysis has demonstrated that the ward is a more interrelated system than would be revealed through relying solely upon the commonly employed fragmented procedures of the past. Through the examination of the nurses' conceptualisations of the ward across a range of different design types, it will be possible to demonstrate the impact of various design characteristics on the structure of the proposed model.

The literature described in this section suggests that nurses are an extremely good source of information with respect to the evaluation of the design of the wards. They have a well articulated wholistic view of the ward which is closely linked to their activities but also includes the activities and feelings of the patients. The literature also indicates that a close relationship exists between the characteristics of the physical design and the ease with which nurses can carry out nursing care. This necessity for a close fit between nursing care and ward design suggests that developments in nursing policy will have great design implications. For example, if early patient ambulation were seriously implemented, as suggested by Roper (1976) nursing care would no longer be at the bedside but at the patient's side. The implications for the nursing profession is a change of emphasis from administering angel, to advisor and teacher. Such a change in role would facilitate the two major concerns of the patient discussed in the previous section, that of increased contact with the staff and greater independence. Moving away from a 'technological fix' approach to a more educationally oriented system of patient care would require a very supportive design. The review of the history and development of ward designs has demonstrated a responsiveness to changing policies. What is needed now is a clearer understanding of what active implementation of policies such as early ambulation would mean for the role of the nurse and of the patient, and what aspects of ward design would best support these redefined user roles.

CONCLUSION

Of all the environments considered in this book, the one for which the term therapeutic is most obviously appropriate is that provided by the acute general hospital. Here it would seem that the medical processes of healing and the nursing activities of caring, combine to provide a setting within which people are to be treated and cured. However, this is an orientation towards therapy which has its roots deep in the profession of medicine, and which can be characterised as derived from the 'medical model'. In evaluating acute general hospitals, then, an implicit evaluation is also being made of the medical model on which they are founded and of the adequacy of the physical form in facilitating the objectives of medical processes.

The review of evaluations of hospitals presented in this chapter has helped to pin-point many of the weaknesses of the medical model and the consequent deficiencies in the design of hospital buildings. It has been argued that in particular the reliance on technology to cure (the 'technological fix), rather than focussing on self-help, education and prevention, has set in motion an approach to hospital design which can at times owe more to factory production processes than to healing and caring for patients. It has further been demonstrated that a fragmentation of the organisation of hospitals and a great divergence of viewpoints about hospital design, between the different professions and levels of the organisational hierarchy, has been encouraged by the medical/technical emphases of the modern hospital.

A spiral of reliance on new procedures and their associated technology, with increasing fragmentation in conceptions and evaluations is implied by the studies reviewed. Furthermore, the patient's voice would appear to be increasingly difficult to hear and increasingly out of key with the fugue of professional opinions. It is argued that the design of hospitals can be one aspect which could help to harmonise the variety of viewpoints and at least slow the escalation of the spiral. However, in order to do this the variety of viewpoints will need to be incorporated in the design process. The literature reviewed in this chapter indicates that post-design evaluation can be harnessed readily to this objective.

REFERENCES

ALKIN, G. (1971) Thoughts on Hospitals, London. 13, 20, 32.
Taken from: Nuffield Provincial Hospitals Trust (1955),
Studies in the Functions and Design of Hospitals, Oxford
University Press and London.

BURTON, I., KATES, R. W., and WHITE, J. F. (1968) 'The Human
Ecology of Extreme Geophysical Events', Natural Hazard
Research Working Paper No. 1, Department of Geography,
University of Toronto.

CANTER, D. (1972) 'Royal Hospital for Sick Children: A
Psychological Analysis', Architects Journal, 6th
September, pp 525-564.

CANTER, D. (1977) 'Children in Hospital: A facet theory
approach to person/place synomorphy', Journal of
Architectural Research, 6/2, August.

CARTWRIGHT, A. (1964) 'Human Relations and Hospital Care',
Routledge and Kegan Paul, London.

COSER, R. (1958) 'Authority and Decision-Making in a
Hospital: A comparative analysis', American Sociology
Review, 23, February, pp 57-63.

EARDLEY, A. and WAKEFIELD, G. (1973) What Patients Think
about the Christie Hospital: A report on 500 interviews,
Manchester: Christie Hospital and Holt Radium Institute,
viii, p 56.

FREEMAN, G. R. and SMALLEY, H. E. (1968) An objective basis
for inpatient nursing unit design, Atlanta, Ga.: School
of Industrial Engineering, Georgia Institute of
Technology, and Medical College of Georgia.

GUTTMAN, L. (1965) 'A faceted definition of intelligence',
in Studies in Psychology, Scripta Hierosolymitana,
Hebrew University, Jerusalem, 14, pp 166-181.

330

GREEN, S. (1974) The Hospital: An organisational analysis,
   Glasgow and London: Blackie.

HAYWARD, J. (1975) Information: A prescription against pain,
   Royal College of Nursing Study of Nursing Care Services,
   London, taken from Wilson-Barnett, 9, 'Patients'
   emotional reactions to hospitalization: an exploratory
   study', in Journal of Advanced Nursing, Vol. 1, 1976.

HICKS, D. (1976) The Management of 120-Bed Clinical Nursing
   Units: an account of research carried out in the five
   years 1970-1974, Part 3, Wessex Regional Health Authority.

HOWARD, G. (1971) An Account of the Principal Lazarettes in
   Europe...with Further Observations on...Hospitals,
   London, 131, 135, 141, taken from Nuffield Provincial
   Hospitals Trust (1955), Studies in the Function and
   Design of Hospitals, London: Oxford University Press.

LIPPERT, S. (1971) 'Travel in Nursing Unit', in Hospital
   Design Evaluation: An interdisciplinary approach,
   H. Field, J. Hanson, C. Karalis, National Technical
   Information Service, Springfield, Va.

NIGHTINGALE, F. (1863) Notes on Hospitals, London, 53, 62.

NUFFIELD PROVINCIAL HOSPITALS TRUST (1953) The Work of Nurses
   in Hospital Wards, London, 92, 94.

NUFFIELD PROVINCIAL HOSPITALS TRUST (1955) Studies in the
   Function and Design of Hospitals, London: Oxford
   University Press.

NUFFIELD FOUNDATION, DIVISION FOR ARCHITECTURAL STUDIES (1962)
   'Nuffield House, Musgrave Park Hospital, Belfast', London:
   Nuffield Foundation.

NOAKES, A. (1971) 'Trends in Ward Planning, 1961-71: New
   policies, new plans and changing shapes', in British
   Ward Design and Equipment Supplement to Hospital
   Management, May/June.

O'LEARY, P. (1973) 'A New Approach to Design-in-Use Evaluation in Hospitals', Hospital Development, September/October.

RAPHAEL, W. (1965) 'If I could alter one thing...', Mental Health, April.

RAPHAEL, W. (1967) 'Do we know what the patients think? A survey comparing the views of patients, staff and committee members', in Int. Nurs. Stud., Vol. 4, pp 209-223, Great Britain: Pergamon Press.

RAPHAEL, W. (1969) Patients and their Hospitals, 2nd Edition, London: King Edwards Fund.

ROPER, N. (1976) 'An Image of Nursing for the 1970s', in Nursing Times, London, April 29, Vol. 72, No. 17, and May 6th, Vol. 72, No. 18, occasional papers.

ROSENGREN, W. R., and DEVAULT, S. (1963) 'The Sociology of Time and Space in an Obstetrical Hospital', in The Hospital in Modern Society, (Ed. E. Freidson), London: The Free Press of Glencoe.

SEARS, D. and AULD, R. (1976) Human Valuation of Complex Environments, Joint Unit for Planning Research, University College, London, and London School of Economics.

STACEY, M. (1977) 'Concepts of Health and Illness: A working paper on the concepts and their relevance for research, in Health and Health Policy: Priorities for research, the report of an advisory panel to the Research Initiatives Board, Social Sciences Research Council, May.

STONE, P. (1976) 'The Heroic Years' in The Architects Journal, 15th December.

STURDAVANT, M. (1960) Comparisons of intensive nursing service in a circular and a rectangular unit, American Hospital Association, Chicago, Ill.

THOMPSON, G. D. (Principal investigator) (1959) Yale studies
of hospital function and design, U.S. Public Health
Service Grant W53.

TRANTER, R. (1969) The Hospital: An investigation into
comfort conditions and patient satisfaction in ward
design, unpublished Ph.D. Dissertation, University of
Wales Institute of Science and Technology.

TRITES, D., GALBRAITH, F., STURDAVANT, M. and LECKWORT, J.
(1970) 'Influence of Nursing-Unit Design on the
Activities and Subjective Feelings of Nursing Personnel',
in Environment and Behavior, Vol. 2, No. 3.

WATERS, A. and MACINTYRE, I. M. C. (1977) Attitudes and
criticisms of surgical in-patients, in The Practitioner,
Vol. 218.

WILSON-BARNETT, J. (1976) 'Patients' emotional reactions to
hospitalization: An exploratory study', in Journal of
Advanced Nursing, Vol. 1, pp 351-358.

Creating Therapeutic Environments

SANDRA AND DAVID CANTER

Institutions, and much implied by that term cannot be planned away. This is graphically illustrated by Rivlin and Wolfe's follow-up of a supposedly novel solution to a psychiatric facility for children. They found that the conventions of the organisation took over and to a large extent neutralised any far sightedness which might have been present in the original design and building. In the different area of provision for mentally retarded children, Mazis and Canter demonstrated that simply reducing the size of a facility and providing it with more domestic accoutrements will not necessarily counteract its becoming institution oriented so long as it is organisationally part of a National Health Service. Whenever a provision for separate groups in the community is identified; whenever distinct locations are regarded as being necessary to provide therapeutic facilities for specific individuals, there will always be a strong possibility of these provisions generating an environment which, whilst supporting administrative wishes, are nonetheless counter-therapeutic.

Furthermore, although radical solutions may contain many answers to this destructive potential of institutions, the very scale and administrative complexity of modern health and welfare provisions will ensure that radical solutions will only nibble at the root causes where systematic solutions, although less attention catching, may well have long term effects which are very dramatic.

In other words, we are arguing that the potential for great improvement in therapeutic settings is available, provided the changes which are made are done so in the knowledge of the complexity of the processes which they are housing, and of the complexity of the administrative framework which has to accommodate them.

Innovations, focused on a particular aspect of the therapeutic setting, will continue to be found to be unsuccessful in the long term, because of the few issues they consider. No matter how original the main impetus of the new therapeutic stance, it will only succeed by being elaborated within a framework which takes the total context into account.

In creating therapeutic environments, then, there are a number of related contributions which together must be effective, and which all too often are lacking. In brief, the components of a successful setting are: (a) attitudes, (b) organisation, and (c) facilities. The actual physical environment itself is not a panacea. Nonetheless, it is apparent that in many situations the mere presence of a distinct environment may be counter-productive to the goals of therapy. Richer's study, for example, demonstrates that by putting autistic children into a special setting it is likely to put in motion a series of actions and reactions which are far less conducive to the children's eventual effective development than is putting them into a conventional school situation.

It has been shown repeatedly in this book that any design solution can only be effective if it relates to a particular context. Therefore, general proposed design solutions cannot be presented. What can be presented are key questions which the administrator or designer must ask of his design/management team. Some possible answers to these questions relevant to the reader's particular context will be found in the earlier pages of this book. However, it is important to emphasise that such questions can only be asked when there is a clear statement of the aims, or goals which the facility is being designed to meet. Ideally, these goals should be ones agreed on by all those involved in designing, administering and using the facility. This is an argument which has a relevance for all buildings. It implies the identification of the activities which it is wished to encourage in order to achieve the organisational goals, and then a specification of environments necessary for the effective pursuance of those activities.

We do not underestimate the frequent difficulties an institution will have in coming to an agreement about its goals and activities. Nonetheless, we are optimistic that by considering the physical environment it is more likely

that an agreement may be reached than about many other
aspects of therapy, where the different professional perspectives can create barriers to discussion. Furthermore,
once the agreement has been reached on physical matters
agreement on other issues may follow more readily.

One of the first questions for the policy maker is:

1. "Is a special environment necessary?"

The particular nature of the deficit of the individuals
which needs to be assisted by the process of therapy will,
in part, determine the answer to this question. It may
well be that conventional facilities, for people who are
not identified as being in need of help, may be deemed
inappropriate for the client group being considered. For
example, putting partially sighted children into a conventional play situation may be far too dangerous for them
and too disturbing for other children. This is certainly
open for discussion, but the example given by Wolff, of an
adventure playground for handicapped children, does illustrate the great value that can be achieved by these children
from a particular setting. There is the open question as
to whether other children without any handicap would also
benefit from such an exciting play facility. However, even
if non-handicapped children would benefit from such a
facility, there is no reason against providing one which
will be geared to the particular use of those who do not
normally have such an opportunity for play. A notion which
reflects the 'enhancement model' discussed in the opening
Chapter.

It is clearly the case that physical provisions can
facilitate many therapeutic processes. If certain types of
spaces are not available, particular equipment, or ready
movement between provisions, then the processes which an
organisation is trying to generate may be severely hampered.
However, if the attitudes of the individuals in the institution are inappropriate, or if the structure and rules of
the organisation itself makes the carrying out of certain
activities difficult or impossible then no amount of physical
facilities will generate the therapeutic processes.

Having presented this caveat there is one curious aspect
of the physical environment which is emerging from the research reported and which provides another question which the
administrator can ask himself.

2. "Can therapeutic processes be set in motion by changes in the physical surroundings?"

The argument here is that it is frequently possible to get agreement about physical changes where it is difficult to get agreement about organisational or social changes. There seems to be a sense in which people are not threatened with the implications of physical changes where they are very threatened with the implications of changing their own activities or relationships with others. Discussions of physical modifications, of course, do frequently revolve around their cost implications. Even though these costs are taken from some public purse the calculations are not usually carried through to the extent that the saving to the public purse in terms of increased numbers of people being returned to the community would bring.

A corollary of the argument that environmental flexibility is typically greater than organisational flexibility is that organisational goals may frequently be undermined by physical modifications. Again, Rivlin and Wolff point to the locking of doors and other minor modifications of the way the physical environment could be used, which grew to have major implications about the type of organisation which was being housed. Gunzburg and Gunzburg cite many individual examples of the way in which general processes of normalisation are being inhibited by physical modifications. This points to another question that the administrator and policy maker must ask themselves:

3. "Are there aspects of the therapeutic process which are being undermined by the designation, utilisation or modification of spaces?

By referring to designation and utilisation as well as modification we are highlighting the fact that it is difficult to disentangle the organisational prerequisites of what a space is for from the actual physical arrangement of that space. The clearest example of this type of situation is that studied in detail by Halohan. Typically, the conventional layout of furniture around the edge of a room, in a sociofugal pattern, is specifically arranged by the cleaning staff who have little idea as to what the room is to be used for. A further example is that illustrated by Sime and Sime, but found in many aspects of the literature. This is the use of spaces as distinctly staff locations and the implicit or explicit removal of patients from those spaces, even though the policy of the organisation may outlaw such obvious distinctions between staff and clients.

When we consider the organisational concomitants of physical form one of the most apparent relationships is to the scale of the organisation. The problems described so graphically by Sommer and Kroll can be seen as part of the problem of organisational size. Mazis and Canter also illustrate in the different setting of homes for mentally retarded children the deficiencies of organisations which can be attributed directly to their size. The policy maker considering the provision of new physical facilities, as a consequence, should ask himself the question:

4. "Does the provision of this facility in this location tend to make it part of a larger setting or does it help to establish it as a smaller unit?"

Clearly, location alone will not determine these features. But a location which facilitates a link with the community such as that discussed in a number of papers, is less likely to be absorbed and treated as part of one monolithic institution than a location which places that facility in such an isolated context that it can only have contact with a nearby large institution. There can, of course, be benefits of scale. Sime and Sime point out the advantages of their forensic unit being based in the grounds of a hospital for mentally retarded patients. Kenny and Canter also illustrate the range of issues which must be considered when dealing with the size of a unit, such as a hospital ward, within a larger unit. It may well often be the case that it is only possible to achieve a number of smaller units provided there is enough of them to make the total scheme viable. Nonetheless, the issue of scale is clearly an area in which administrators are led, by the increased ease of their own processes, towards the agglomeration of larger and larger units.

The therapist wishes for smaller units in which many of the benefits of close interaction between the various individuals can be obtained. However, at the present time it is not clear when any small unit is, in effect, part of a larger unit, or when it can operate relatively independently and thus, obtain the benefits of its smaller size. It is unlikely that there will be one single answer to this issue. The particular client group needs to be carefully considered and the resources on which it must draw. Richer's example of using an ordinary school for children as a setting in which to absorb modified facilities for autistic children, and the example of Sime and Sime for the absorption of forensic cases, both point to the potential advantages to the smaller unit of being absorbed into a more conventional

facility which lacks its own stigma. On the other hand,
when dealing with facilities which encompass so many individuals that they can develop a characteristic style and mode
of operation of their own, such as the homes for mentally
retarded children, it appears that there is a penalty to
be paid for accommodating these facilities in large units.

One aspect of scale which also has design concomitants
is that of autonomy. The question the administrator can put
to himself here is:

5. "Does this facility have the administrative autonomy
which is most effective for stimulating staff attitudes
towards therapeutic processes?"

Clearly a unit which is an integrated part of a larger
setting is less likely to develop its own autonomy than one
placed in a separate, distinct building. Most policy makers
are afraid of autonomy being abused. Because institutions
are typically the responsibility of some public domain and
accountability is frequently felt to be necessary, senior
administrators feel that their heads will roll if a local
institution does not live up to public scrutiny. In order
to safeguard themselves against this possibility they take
more of the control of the organisation onto themselves.
However, as Kushlick (quoted in the opening chapter of this
book) has so elegantly pointed out, once this distant authority is in control it can only check the processes carried
out in the institution on some simple or short visit basis.
It can observe how clean an institution is, or whether
certain guidelines about activities are being followed
through. It cannot supervise, in the normal course of
events, the day to day interactions between patients and
staff. The staff in their turn, feel the need to keep the
patients under control so that they can demonstrate that
they are carrying out things according to the master plan.
The result here is frequently the moulding of patients to
fit the administrative policy. Lipman and Slater's proposal
for a home for old people is an attempt to counteract this
trend by a design solution. By providing a facility in
which the contact between staff and residents is kept as
distant as possible, they feel the likelihood of patients
having their behaviour modified to fit in with staff requirements and to increase the patients' dependency on staff,
is reduced. Beyond this attempt to shape the environment
so that the processes of autonomy both for staff and for
clients can be increased there is the procedure which Sommer
and Kroll so readily illustrate. This is the attempt to
set in motion regular appraisal of the facility so that

central administrators can have a clear picture of what it
is they are managing. Throughout these readings there are
a number of examples of the procedures available to them.
This leads to the further question which the administrator
may ask himself:

6. "Are there some appraisal processes which we ought to
set in motion in order to find out clearly what is the nature
of our current environmental estate?"

The approach of Rivlin and Wolff of following up facilities over time does not lend itself to ready administrative
use. However, if it is done in association with other
procedures it can prove very valuable. Procedures more
directly linked to a short visit are those illustrated by
Mazis and Canter and by Sommer and Kroll. Both of these
provide indications of short, ready to use, scales which can
quickly provide a good picture of a facility. Putting
these scales together with observational strategies such as
those employed by Rivlin and Wolff and by Sime and Sime
show that there is a great range of tried and tested procedures which can produce very useful information.

One of the issues that clearly needs to be explored
when assessing the state of any facility may be related to
the recurrent theme of the potency of the 'medical model'.
Observations can quickly reveal whether the pattern of user
descriptions of the facility or of activities carried out
within it, owe more to what would be expected of a surgical
ward in a hospital than to other sorts of therapeutic setting.
It is not that high levels of cleanliness or very specific
routines of the use of facilities, nor even the presence of
nurses' stations or the control of movement of residents
about the facility, all illustrated in a number of papers,
are of themselves necessarily counter therapeutic. It is
that there is a growing indication that where such clearly
medically oriented aspects occur there is a strong likelihood
that many other aspects of an inappropriate medical model
can be found, notably a lack of concern for the experiences
of the clients as people, rather than patients. Notes of
such details then can act as quick guides to the general
approach of a facility and the ready question of whether it
is as effective as it might be. It is clear that in many
situations the clean pristine ward in which individuals are
only allowed to sleep may be quite against the provisions
appropriate to a therapeutic community.

Putting the issue of the medical orientedness of an
institution together with the points of autonomy and scale
to which we have already referred leads to a further

recurring design aspect. An aspect to which almost all
authors make some reference throughout these papers. In
summary, it can be referred to as the need to pay attention
to the details. To convert this into a question which the
administrator should ask himself we can say:

7. "Are the details of the provisions in the physical setting
appropriate for the goals of that setting?"

To provide some more examples of this, one can ask if
there are the bits and pieces around which would be common
in many private homes and which are important for parents
and children alike to use and play with. The availability
of cutlery or the location of the kitchens, the easy access
to rooms for informal use, the colouring of walls and doors
to remove disorientation, the concern for transport systems
as well as what happens when you reach a place, all these
details have been shown to have potentially great significance for residents in instutitions. All too often the
master plan of a design is sketched out in terms of blank
boxes with number of patients written in and broad relationships established. Buildings, it would seem, are still
designed from the outside inwards; frequently the inside is
left as something of an afterthought. Of course, attention
must be given to the size and relationship of buildings,
but it is the details of what is available within those
buildings and what use can be made of what is available,
which is a major contribution which the environment can make
to the therapeutic process. It is in this area also that
the clients themselves can be involved in both decisions
about and changing of details of the environment. This very
process of deciding and changing can be of therapeutic value
in itself.

Following through all of the questions presented above
implies that some sequence of changes is liable to be set
in motion. It must be emphasised that the particular nature
of the facilities being considered may give quite different
answers to the questions posed. The consensus which is
apparent throughout the papers in this book perhaps suggest
that we are beginning to explore this broad area but that,
again, many of the implications of these explorations have
not been followed through. However, there is one implication
of all these potentials for change which is most directly
illustrated by the paper by Halohan. This is the need for
consultation to take place throughout any process of change.
In one sense this recommendation for consultation is an
aspect of the general issue of the benefit provided by autonomy. For people to make most effective use of their

facilities it is necessary that they be involved directly
in any modifications which take place to them, or indeed,
in the initial development of them. The properties of the
private facilities which Mazis and Canter found, was in part
due to the influence which the local people could have over
the provisions in which they were housed. Similarly, the
aspects of normalisation to which Gunzburg and Gunzburg
refer, is much more readily available when the staff and
residents can have control over the decisions relating to
their own environment. In essence, Lipman and Slater's
proposal is a way of enabling the residents themselves to
have more possibility for autonomy and control over any
small changes they may wish to introduce into their own
settings. To return to Halohan's paper again, the fact that
some groups of staff initially neutralised his modifications
because they had not been consulted about the proposed
changes, is an illustration of how a group within an organisation can have a destructive effect no matter what environmental changes are instituted.

We have put forward our proposals in the form of questions which policy makers and administrators should ask
themselves. This is not in an attempt to avoid making
specific recommendations but in the belief that any recommendation must be specific to a particular context. By
identifying the issues which the administrator must satisfy
himself on for a given context, we believe that considerable
improvements can take place. If he decides to answer these
questions in ways which may be different from the trend
implied in the preceding pages then that clearly is the
administrator's prerogative. Nonetheless, it is a prerogative which can be acted on openly in relation to a particular
situation. By bringing out into the open the key points for
discussion we are helping to remove what Sommer, in the
context of prisons, demonstrates to be one of the major
problems. This is what he calls paeleologic. A type of
prehistoric argument that has its roots in feelings and is
relatively impervious to logical analysis. By bringing
matters into open discussion and identifying clearly the
questions which must be answered it is much more difficult
for paeleologic to survive. We are not pretending that the
design of therapeutic environments is an easy task nor one
that can be resolved with a few bold strokes. However, we
are firm believers in the optimism apparent in a systematic
approach.

The great advantage of an organic system is that when
certain changes have been introduced they can grow and develop
and find their way through the whole system. If nurtured
appropriately they can contribute to a more positive era in
therapeutic environments.

342

REFERENCE

SOMMER, R. (1977) <u>The end of imprisonment</u>, Oxford University Press.

Author Index

The Editors are grateful to Peter Reid for compiling the indices.

Subject Index

350